Praise for

# BUTT SERIOUSLY

"Anal sex is hard to talk about—even people who enjoy it sometimes feel uncomfortable around the topic. Dr. Goldstein's affirming, approachable, and deeply informed, user-friendly advice is the best thing to happen to anal sex since lube was invented. I can't recommend this book highly enough."

—Dan Savage, author of *Savage Love* and host of *Savage Lovecast*

"If you want to learn about anal play, sex, and pleasure, *Butt Seriously* is everything you ever wanted. Dr. Evan Goldstein has now written the definitive guide on how to prepare for anal, what to do if things go wrong, and my favorite…anal myths we can now let go of! Informed by research but written with wit and warmth, this is the book I'll now be recommending to anyone ready to make anal pleasure a part of their life."

—Emily Morse, host of the *Sex with Emily* podcast, doctor of human sexuality, and author of *Smart Sex: How to Boost Your Sex IQ and Own Your Pleasure*

"No but(t)s about it, Evan Goldstein has written a definitive, personable, and sorely needed guide to all things anal!"

—Ian Kerner, PhD, LMFT, *New York Times* bestselling author of *She Comes First*

"If you Google 'anal sex tips,' you'll see dozens of articles with the same three recommendations: breathe, use lots of lube, and go slowly... but that's it. When you start having anal sex, you'll have about a hundred more questions on preparation, dilation, aftercare, enhancing pleasure, et cetera. And you won't be able to find those answers anywhere online. Unless you specifically see a gay sexual-health doctor, odds are your health-care provider won't have answers, either. *Butt Seriously* answers every single damn question you could have about anal play. It is by far the most thorough manual on anal sex, and Dr. Goldstein approaches the topic in the most sex-positive, shame-free manner that encourages everyone to explore the wonders of their backdoor."

—Anal aficionado Zachary Zane, author of
*Boyslut: A Memoir and Manifesto*

"*Butt Seriously* is a serious book about butts. Goldstein offers a comprehensive and accessible guide to the ins and outs of anal play. Shining a light on topics that are almost completely neglected in traditional sex ed, this book empowers readers with the knowledge they need to take control of their sexual health and pleasure from the bottom up."

—Justin J. Lehmiller, PhD, host of the *Sex and Psychology*
podcast and author of *Tell Me What You Want*

"*Butt Seriously* brings both lightness and depth to an often-taboo topic. A nonjudgmental and incredibly informative read, this book is perfect for anyone who wants to get their peach in top working order to experience and give pleasure with more ease."

—Rae McDaniel, certified sex therapist,
author of *Gender Magic*

"Written by a renowned expert and anal sex guru, this is the only book you need for information that's accurate but also sex positive. Anal health is an important part of sexual health, but more importantly a huge part of sexual expression. Avoiding anal is avoiding pleasure—this book dispels myths, discusses important anatomy, and how to fix problems to reduce butt anxiety and build more sexual confidence."

—Chris Donaghue, PhD, LCSW, CST

"Finally, a complete guide to one of our most important body parts."

—Nichole Klatt, PhD, professor and division chief of Surgical Outcomes and Precision Medicine Research, University of Minnesota Department of Surgery

# BUTT
## SERIOUSLY

# BUTT
# SERIOUSLY

The Definitive Guide to
Anal Health, Pleasure, and
Everything In Between

## DR. EVAN GOLDSTEIN

balance

NEW YORK  BOSTON

Copyright © 2024 by Evan Goldstein

Cover design by Jim Datz
Front cover photograph © Chiccododifc/Shutterstock
Back cover photograph © Sarkao/Shutterstock
Cover copyright © 2024 by Hachette Book Group, Inc.

Hachette Book Group supports the right to free expression and the value of copyright. The purpose of copyright is to encourage writers and artists to produce the creative works that enrich our culture.

The scanning, uploading, and distribution of this book without permission is a theft of the author's intellectual property. If you would like permission to use material from the book (other than for review purposes), please contact permissions@hbgusa.com. Thank you for your support of the author's rights.

Balance
Hachette Book Group
1290 Avenue of the Americas
New York, NY 10104
GCP-Balance.com
@GCPBalance

First edition: May 2024

Balance is an imprint of Grand Central Publishing. The Balance name and logo are registered trademarks of Hachette Book Group, Inc.

The publisher is not responsible for websites (or their content) that are not owned by the publisher.

Balance books may be purchased in bulk for business, educational, or promotional use. For information, please contact your local bookseller or the Hachette Book Group Special Markets Department at special.markets@hbgusa.com.

Illustrations by Boyking

Library of Congress Control Number: 2024931385

ISBNs: 9781538757475 (trade paperback), 9781538757482 (ebook)

Printed in the United States of America

LSC-C

Printing 1, 2024

*Dedicated to my partner, Andy, and our two beautiful boys,*
*Phoenix and Sebastian.*
*None of this would have been possible without the sacrifices*
*overcome by our community.*

*We have two lives, and the second begins when we realize we only have one.*

—Confucius

# Contents

## PART I:
## THE BARE BASICS

## PART II:
## GOING ALL IN

# PART III:
# AFTERCARE

# PART I

# THE BARE BASICS

# CHAPTER 1

# You're Not Alone

"I'm fucked, Doctor Goldstein." Keith, the twenty-one-year-old with a sweet smile sitting across from me in my office, looked like your typical Jersey boy. Like many of the young gay men I'd treated who were raised in supportive, sex-positive environments, he didn't seem embarrassed to be meeting with an anal surgeon. In fact, he radiated positivity. The only thing bumming him out was, well, his bum.

I wasn't the first anal surgeon he'd visited. A few years prior, he'd sought treatment for anal warts, symptoms of a common STI among people who engage in anal sex (though not exclusive to them). His first doctor had successfully removed the warts, but ever since, the slightest pressure in his anus caused him pain. For years, he hadn't been able to take a shit without bleeding, much less enjoy receiving anal sex like he used to. Now he was in a new relationship that felt serious, but the pain and frustration at being unable to fully express himself sexually were taking their toll. So yeah, Keith was fucked, and not the way he wanted to be.

Keith's experience wasn't uncommon. The initial surgery had indeed removed the warts, but in their place had grown delicate scar tissue that had never healed properly, creating a chronic weak spot that would split and tear at the slightest pressure. Fortunately, it was a pretty easy surgical fix, and I had Keith in and out of my operating room within thirty minutes. In short order he no longer dreaded going to the bathroom. But it wasn't just his butt that needed fixing; it was his whole sex life. Here, too, I was happy to help. Over the course of a few monthly visits, my team and I rehabilitated Keith's ass until he was ready to engage sexually again. I only saw him a few times over the next three or four years, but each time, he was beaming. That new relationship had turned out to be the love of his life. He was well and truly fucked, he assured me, but in a very, very good way.

When my patient Kara came to see me she was simultaneously raving about and cursing her two young children for ushering her into motherhood with a first-class case of hemorrhoids. She'd been assured that the discomfort and bleeding she experienced in her ass would subside a few months after giving birth, but the kids were now five years and six months old, and exercise and going to the bathroom were still a constant source of pain and concern for her. She was also grossed out by what felt like excess skin growing back there. It wasn't comfortable to wear a G-string anymore. She didn't feel sexy at all, and it was hurting her sex life. Something had to change.

Upon examination, I discovered that Kara did have hemorrhoids, but it was actually an angry anal tear, likely caused by the intense pressure of childbirth, that was causing the majority of her pain and bleeding. One 15-minute procedure and the problem was fixed. For about three months Kara came in for follow-up care, which included learning to use toys to help rehabilitate the anal muscles. Last I spoke to her, she said she finally felt like herself. No longer distracted by her ass, she'd been able to focus on her kids and gain confidence in her new role as a mom. She'd also regained confidence in the bedroom. Getting her sexy back had rekindled her desire for intimacy with her husband, so that even though both were exhausted by midnight diaper changes and the all-consuming needs of young children, their marriage felt stronger than ever.

I make my living dealing with assholes. Usually they're attached to nice people seeking help for a host of common issues causing them pain or embarrassment. Many of my patients are young and LGBTQ+, like Keith, needing relief from injuries caused by improperly executed anal sex, or treatment for anal STIs. But I also frequently see people of all genders and sexual orientations, like Kara, who are seeking help for conditions caused by constipation, childbirth, and even poor weightlifting techniques. I see damage from overwiping with rough toilet paper, or rashes or fungal or bacterial irritations caused by overuse of wet wipes. I meet people suffering from hemorrhoids, who are scared when they see unexplained blood in the toilet bowl. I talk to patients who just don't feel sexy because of unwanted hair or irregular pigmentation. And their sex lives suffer as much as their bodies and confidence. Ultimately, one thing seems to be universally true: No one feels happy, healthy, or beautiful if their ass isn't happy, healthy, and beautiful. So that's what I do—give people their happiness, health, and self-confidence back, one butt at a time.

Welcome to the zero-judgment zone, where no topics are off-limits, and all are welcome.

If you have a penis, have a seat. If you have a vagina, get comfortable. If you're trans or even just thinking about transitioning, genderqueer, nonbinary, or intersex, make yourself at home. If you have no clue where you fall on the sexual orientation or gender identity spectrum, there is space for you here. Because whether you're gay or straight, bi or pan, cis, trans, nonbinary, or anything and everything we haven't thought of or for which we don't yet have the language, *everyone* has an asshole, and too few people know how to treat or use it right. That's tragic for two reasons. One, the anus is a fundamental organ that needs as much attention and preventative care as any other, and two, it can be a powerful erogenous zone, offering access to the kind of joyful, sweaty, exhilarating sex that everyone who desires it should get to enjoy, and enjoy often.

Which isn't to say people aren't giving it their best shot! When my team surveyed a cohort of sexually active American adults—including about their anal sex experiences, we found that 72 percent had tried either bottoming (receiving anal sex) or topping (penetrating). One in four has tried both. Among gay men, 94 percent have tried bottoming, 91 percent have topped, and 85 percent have tried both. It's not just the fresh young things who are interested in anal, either. Yes, 70 percent of Gen Z has tried some form of anal sex, but so has 70 percent of Gen X and 74 percent of Millennials.[1] Unfortunately, many who've tried anal and no longer engage in it cite pain as a deterrent, and fear of pain is a primary reason why many others have said they won't even consider it. Meanwhile, "anal" consistently lands in the top ten searched terms on the world's biggest porn site.[2]

What does this mean? It means that a lot of people are engaging anally, and a lot more want to. Every day, I meet people who feel like they're missing out on an important piece of sexual intimacy and expression because they're too scared to admit they want it up the butt, or because they're self-conscious about the aesthetics of their ass, or because the sex is painful, or because they just can't get their body to do what they want it to do. They can Google, but most of the information on the internet is wildly unhelpful or even wrong. Fear of pain keeps a whole other population from even trying. That's a tragedy! Because anal sex and anal play, when done right, is HOT. More people deserve to know how good it can be, and for those already engaging, how much better they can make it.

## ANAL'S ON THE RISE

While gay men represent the largest group that engages in anal sex—props to Lil Nas X for announcing himself as a power bottom at the end of 2021—interest in anal has been gaining momentum across gay and straight communities for years, in large part because of its normalization in pop culture. In 1998, as *Sex and the City*'s Charlotte debated becoming "up-the-butt-girl," her best friend Samantha assured her it was wonderful. In 2001, Ben and McKinley's passionate anal tryst in *Wet Hot American Summer* was one of the few legit tender moments in the whole film. In 2014, Paxton from *How to Get Away with Murder* murmured that a legal intern "did this thing to my ass that made my eyes water." We've witnessed Marnie, bent over a kitchen sink in the fourth season premiere of *Girls*, moan with pleasure while receiving analingus, and Armond and Dillon's workplace rimming session in the first season of *The White Lotus* had gay

Twitter alternately cheering and clamoring to step in as the show's "ass eating consultant."[3] (*The White Lotus* followed up by depicting penetrative anal sex in Season Two.) *Broad City*'s Abbi donned a bright green strap-on dildo to penetrate her new boyfriend, and Ryan Reynolds got it up the butt in *Deadpool*. From movies to music to mainstream magazine articles, America has increasingly been exposed to positive images of and references to anal sex. Why *wouldn't* you want to try it?

The problem is that while entertaining, most of these depictions make it seem like anyone can have a great anal experience at a moment's notice. In reality, unless you know what you're doing, that's just not the case. If you've ever felt confused, disappointed, or disillusioned in your quest to have great anal sex, you're not alone. Most people have a tough time getting the hang of it, and unfortunately, it isn't the kind of thing where practice inevitably makes perfect. If you continue on unaware of your or your partner's particular anatomical structure and what it takes to get the body in shape to deliver and receive the sex you desire, you're more than likely destined for disappointment. And until now, it was hard to find a teacher.

There's a hole in the proctological world. Most times, I'm a patient's last stop after a long, frustrating search for someone who understands them. Many women will start out trying to talk to gynecologists, who promptly redirect them toward anal specialists. People who are injured or in pain will bounce from one ineffective treatment to another, or wait months for appointments with anal doctors at elite medical institutions. They go in hoping that once they're treated they'll also get insight into how to address their sexual needs, only to discover that most ass specialists are uncomfortable discussing how to use it for sex or sexiness. Traditionally, anal doctors have considered a treatment successful if it results in regular, pain-free bowel movements and a clean bill of anal health. But if someone believes they could achieve great pleasure in taking things up the butt, and they find that no matter what they try they can't get the mechanics to work, to me, no matter how satisfying your poops are, that's not a success! I've found that the benchmarks of the system, the goals of the practitioner, and the needs of the community are too often misaligned. It's a travesty that the anal medical field has failed to develop a formal sexual-wellness educational protocol. That's why I developed my own.

This country does a piss-poor job of educating people about their bodies, their reproductive organs, and baby-making sex; education about the anus is almost nonexistent. Few people know where to turn for expert, reliable information, guidance, and advice. Until now, they've mostly had to rely on porn, Reddit, and experimentation to figure out how to top, bottom, or engage in any other type of anal play, which is why so many people who do try anal get hurt. That's why I wrote this book. It's the first medically sound, comprehensive, entertaining guide that will teach you everything you need to know about how to keep your ass healthy, beautiful, and ready to take you to the heights of sexual bliss. It's the kind of resource I wish I'd had access to a long time ago.

## PHYSICIAN, HEAL THYSELF

Before I was a gay anal surgeon catering to and championing the LGBTQ+ community of New York City, I was a general surgical resident heading to a cardiothoracic fellowship, living in suburban Long Island, married to a woman. While in medical school, I ate poorly, barely slept, and spent my days stressed as hell. I treated my body like crap, and my crap treated me accordingly, eventually making me so constipated I developed an anal tear that made every bowel movement feel like a raccoon had clawed its way up my ass. It got so bad I finally sought medical help. I was thinking they'd give me some kind of stool softeners, suppositories, or lotions; instead, I was told that the problem was so severe I needed surgery. The doctor cleaned up the tear and performed a partial sphincterotomy, a procedure in which one of the sphincter muscles is cut to release tension and increase blood flow around the wound, which allows the tear to resolve. I was studying to heal the ticker, not the tail. There was no way for me to know I'd just undergone a procedure that could negatively affect me for the rest of my life.

The surgery was a success, sort of. If I watched what I ate and used proper pooping technique (yes, there is one, and you'll learn more about it in chapter 4). I could go weeks without pain, but inevitably I'd stop being as careful as I should and the tear would reopen, though never as severely as pre-surgery. It was uncomfortable, but bearable. Just a thing I'd have to learn to live with.

It wasn't until I came out as gay that the bigger ramification of that pain in the butt revealed itself. I hadn't yet tried bottoming and it seemed to me bottoms were having a lot of fun, so I wanted to try it with my new partner, Andy. The mechanics seemed simple, so one day, spur of the moment, I went bottoms up. And it hurt. I mean, like a sonofabitch. Not only were Andy and I inexperienced and unaware that your poor asshole can't just stretch from zero to balls-deep without any prep, but that old wound announced loud and clear that my ass had built-in limits. No bottoming for me.

I was like a lot of the patients who walk through my door today—confused, frustrated, and completely self-educated, which means much of what I thought I was doing right was absolutely wrong. Now for me, accepting that I couldn't engage anally because I'd never healed properly wasn't the end of the world, and my partner was understanding. But for some who think of themselves as bottoms and can't perform the way they want to, or can't fulfill the desires they crave—at least without pain—it can be a real confidence buster. It's no better for tops, whose experience is usually heightened by their partners' enjoyment and gratification, and dampened when they don't. In addition, many tops are tops either because it hurts too much for them to bottom, or they're afraid of the stigma and worry bottoming will hurt their image or sense of masculinity. Not knowing enough about our bodies and how to maximize their pleasure is a problem that can undermine our sex life and relationships as surely as less-taboo issues like low libido, premature ejaculation, or painful vaginal intercourse.

I looked around to find who was delivering the kind of medical treatment, particularly surgical treatment, and sexual health advice someone like me needed. The answer was nobody. I called major hospitals and scoured the internet for leads, but the doctors who catered to gay men were still primarily concerned with HIV management, even though successful therapies, medicines, and preventative practices to control HIV lethality and spread had been in use since the mid-1990s. HIV was no longer a death

sentence, yet few medical practitioners seemed ready to acknowledge that the community had more to contend with than just
this one disease. They weren't focusing on sexual issues. Those
who did do anal work, like proctologists and surgeons, were
approaching the butt from a heteronormative standpoint, meaning their goal was to ensure their patients could take regular,
painless shits. They weren't interested in destigmatizing anal sex,
or really even talking about it at all, and they certainly didn't see
any need to address anal aesthetics. There are potential complications when doing any kind of surgery, and most believed that it
was safer to just leave things alone back there, since as far as they
were concerned, no one was going to see it anyway. The fact that
the issue affected your self-confidence or sense of sexiness didn't
matter—except for a lot of people, including me, it did. For those
of us who valued the sexual potential and aesthetics of the ass as
much as its utilitarian function, there was nowhere to go.

I pivoted from thoracic surgery, and Bespoke Surgical was
born. I built the practice as a safe space where people could come
to receive healing without judgment, where they'd be encouraged
to ask questions, where we'd debunk myths and defang taboos,
and celebrate patients' sexual needs and desires, as well as their
aesthetic preferences. As often as possible, I wanted my patients
to be physically able to fulfill their mental and emotional desires.
I wanted to build a learning space where I could teach partners
how to communicate and set the stage for successful relationships. Eventually, I started sharing what I knew not just with my
patients, but with a wider audience through blogs and articles.
Now, when people Googled, "How to engage anally," "Does
anal sex hurt?" or, "Is bleeding after anal sex normal?" they had

access to doctor-led, scientifically accurate information and best practices.

I was featured in national publications like *GQ*, *Men's Health*, *Insider*, *Cosmo*, and *Playboy*, and started getting invited to interviews on podcasts like *Savage Lovecast* and *Sex with Emily*. I was asked to speak everywhere from the Icahn School of Medicine at Mount Sinai Colon and Rectal Conference, to Stimulate, the first national sexual wellness conference, to ButtCon, aka "Comic-con for butts." Word got out that I was someone patients could trust to start the conversations few other doctors were willing to have. Today, I see about ninety patients and perform about six to twelve surgeries per week, and I have a month-long waiting list. In 2019, I launched Future Method, a sexual wellness brand dedicated to developing products and educational content that empower people to properly care for their bodies before, during, and after sex. I could see that too many people were using questionable, unsubstantiated, even harmful products, and decided to develop better, safer tools, toys, and other sexual wellness items backed by rigorous research. Our tagline is "The Science of Sex."

Time passed, my career soared, my relationship with Andy deepened, yet I never stopped wishing that I could bottom. After learning all the ins and outs of the butt, developing my product line, and—this was interesting—walking my own team through one more surgical procedure to rebuild my ass and finally repair the damage caused by the ill-advised sphincterotomy, I found the courage to try again. I took matters into my own hands, so to speak. I injected Botox into my ass (yes, really, and once you read chapter 5 you might, too) and practiced my anal dilation exercises (also covered in chapter 5) and in just a few weeks I'd reached the top of my anal game. My confidence in the effectiveness of our curriculum and treatment protocols lies not only in the positive feedback I get from my patients and the results I witness, but because they worked for me.

## LET'S GET IT ON

I'm a rarity in my field—an anal surgeon with a thriving practice who also takes it up the ass. A doctor who not only understands the LGBTQ+ community, but is a member of it. And I've been where you are, harboring desires, but not knowing how to fulfill them. Thanks to my research and personal experiences as a gay man, I have unparalleled insight not only into the physical issues people face when they wish to enjoy anal play, but the psychological and emotional issues that can get in the way of people engaging successfully and pleasurably. The solutions to most of our problems and the answers to our questions are generally quite simple. What's harder is destigmatizing the conversation and overriding people's insecurities. Patients and practitioners have got to open up, so to speak, so we can start talking about our asses as freely as we do about any other body part.

I wrote this book for you, whether you're a gay married man, a recent divorcee, a young person exploring your sexuality, a hetero who's anal-curious but too nervous to try, or even a mom who wants to spice things up in the bedroom. It's a comprehensive, science-backed yet accessible guide to all things anal, with emphasis on how to achieve your ideal form, function, and fuckability. Whatever stage of anal exploration you're in, whether just getting started or ready to stretch your, um, imagination, it will help you learn how to make whatever experience you're looking for be the best it can be, with takeaways such as:

- Step-by-step instructions for tops and bottoms to successfully engage in and enjoy anal sex, regardless of gender or sexual identity
- A detailed takedown of the anal sex myths used to foster shame, fear, and homophobia
- Individualized guidance for people with prostates or vulvas on accessing their erogenous zones for the most mind-blowing orgasms
- A six-week booty camp to train your ass to comfortably accept almost any kind of penetration
- Everything you need to know to keep your ass healthy, functional, and beautiful, inside and out
- Proper pooping technique for optimal health and keeping your ass primed for good sex
- Anal-sex-friendly diet and nutrition tips to keep sex spontaneous and mess-free
- Recommendations for the most effective sexual techniques, hottest toys, slickest lubes, and other products
- Suggestions for questions you should ask and be asked in a doctor's office, and medical standards you should expect and demand if you engage anally

Everyone and anyone can benefit from the sexual education provided here. Gay men can learn what high standards they should expect from their medical practitioners and how to advocate for themselves. Non-gay men can expand their sexual repertoires.

Straight women can discover a whole new universe of sexual pleasure. No one has been left out.

The book is structured in three parts. Part I is all about setting the stage for success, from introducing you to a community that's much larger and more diverse than you probably ever imagined, to helping you think through your sexual desires and goals, to dissecting and debunking all the garbage myths and misinformation swirling around anal sex and play. You'll also get a robust lesson in anal anatomy. None of this is just nice-to-know stuff—all of your anal pleasure starts with you paying attention here. In Part II, we're going in (but for God's sake, not all at once!), covering advice and techniques for properly preparing the butt to comfortably receive, as well as how to maximize your and your partner's pleasure while minimizing complications.

**TOP TIPS:** Tops, throughout the book, keep an eye out for asides like these filled with Top Tips that highlight how understanding the material in each chapter can ease and enhance your experience. That's not just the bottom's responsibility. It's your job, too. You can help them relax. You can help create a sexy, supportive environment. It's often customary to blame bottoms when things don't go as well as we'd hoped, but the problem is often not with the bottom, but with the top. It can be a letdown to knock at the door and find that your more-than-willing partner can't figure out how to unlock it, but remember, you're the goddamn key. Learn how to use it correctly. With the right knowledge, you can be instrumental in helping partners swing their portals open smoothly and easily. Every new partner has the potential to be the greatest fuck of your life—and who knows, maybe even the greatest relationship of your life. Don't miss out on it because you don't know what you don't know. I'm all about empowering bottoms to ask for what they want and learn what they can get, but I want everyone to get the fruitful sex they desire.

Following the prep protocols and instructions outlined in the book should help prevent injuries in the first place, but if they do occur, Part III is all about what to do, and how to ensure you stay healthy and in great shape for next time. We'll also talk through the daily habits you can adopt and the state-of-the art services available to achieve an aesthetically beautiful asshole. While there's a wide range in people's attitudes to perfectly natural variations in skin, hair, size, and shape, *nothing* about your body is gross or unsightly. Unless *you* decide it is, of course, in which case you'll learn the possible remedies here.

Along the way, you'll be privy to more than a decade's worth of stories and anecdotes from real patients I've met over the course of my career, which should reassure you that whatever questions you have, fears you need to work through, problems you've experienced or kinks you want to indulge, you aren't the first and you won't be the last. Trust me; I've heard and seen it all.

You hold in your hands a cheeky yet authoritative guide to amazing anal sex and better anal health, yet it's about much more than that. It's about going after what you want. It's about improving your relationships. This truth was brought home to me the day I opened my email to find a letter informing me that Keith had been killed in a car accident the day before. Aside from sharing the terrible news, Keith's partner wanted me to know how grateful Keith had been to be my patient, not just because I resolved a medical issue that had been an impediment for too long, but for the advice and guidance I'd shared, which he'd then applied to his relationship with his partner. In the end, Keith's partner wrote, the intimacy I'd enabled them to have allowed them to become closer as a couple. Their time together had been tragically short, but it had been wonderful.

Everyone should have a chance at that kind of sexual fulfillment and completion, whether they're in a monogamous long-term relationship or still hitting the apps. I started my surgical career thinking that I wanted to heal the heart, and though today I cut and stitch at the body's opposite end, indirectly, that's still often what I do. My goal is bigger than teaching as many people as possible everything they need to know about this particular body part. It's to give as many people as possible the opportunity to explore and express their complete selves. With the right training, the extent to which you can expand your sexual potential, so to speak, is likely much higher than you ever imagined. Enjoy the ride!

## CHAPTER 2

# Five Bogus ASSumptions and Other Junk in Our Trunk

I often say that my work with patients is 60 percent functional, 40 percent mental. Yes, I heal people's body parts when they come to me with pain or a problem, but I also frequently find myself having heart-to-heart talks with my patients about learning to trust and love their bodies—sometimes for the first time—and how to let someone else love them, too. Most of us, even those of us who know we love anal, carry a buttload of baggage around it. I see it in my work each day. People embarrassed to admit they'd like to try it. People afraid to embrace their sexuality. People whose sense of masculinity risks being shattered by the realization they crave playing a sexually submissive role. People filled with fear and self-doubt, wondering, *Am I sexy enough? How does my ass look? Am I going to shit on someone if I do this? Am I going to bleed?* The emotional and psychological weight of internalized shame or self-loathing will tank your sex life if you let it.

Where does this weight come from? Ignorance, fear, and homophobia have spurred countless myths around the topic of anal sex, about who does it, and how, and why. They feed absurd ideas that we absorb through cultural norms, peers, inadequate sex education, political misinformation and laws grounded in bigotry and bias, inaccurate Reddit posts, and unrealistic porn. It's insidious, and it piles up. After years of being steeped in these myths, it's no wonder so many of us have a warped, inaccurate view of what anal sex is like, who gets to have it, and whether it can be a "normal" addition to someone's sexual repertoire.

There is absolutely nothing perverse or abnormal about enjoying or wanting anal sex. But it's not enough for me to tell you, you have to believe it, or there's no point reading any further. You can't reap the rewards of the advice in this book if you don't unpack and get rid of any biases, judgment, and self-hatred you've developed as a result of living in a society that stupidly insists on loading anal sex with stigma and making it taboo. If you're willing to examine the myths surrounding anal sex, you'll find that not one holds up under scrutiny. Not one.

For many, that revelation is all it takes to start undoing the negative effects of unnecessary denial, repression, and shame. It's exhilarating. It can be scary. Not everyone is open to it. I had a straight patient who had been experimenting with anal sex, but as the date of his arranged marriage approached, he asked me to surgically tighten his asshole up again so his wife wouldn't suspect he was into anal. I performed the surgery because it's what he wanted, but I kept wondering about a different universe in which he felt he could be honest about the type of sex he liked, and enjoy it with his wife. It's just so sad to know people still choose to live in self-imposed traps of denial and shame rather than embrace who they are. If this is you and you're considering making the leap, I promise there is a large community waiting to catch and celebrate you when you're ready.

In my experience, once people are no longer hung up on fiction, they're excited to explore where the pleasure and power of anal engagement can take them, and far more likely to have consistently good physical and emotional experiences. Learning the truth helps get them out of their head and out of their own way. In the interest of helping you join their ranks, I'm thrilled to have this opportunity to explain why the following most common, harmful myths, five in all, are complete and utter bullshit.

## ASSUMPTION #1: THE ASS ISN'T MEANT FOR PLEASURE

Enjoy your first anal orgasm, then tell me the ass isn't meant for pleasure. On the contrary, it's built for it, no matter whose body it belongs to. The entire region where we engage sexually is loaded with sensitive nerve endings that respond exquisitely to stimulation whether you're coming at them from the front or back, in or out, and organs and glands create multiple intensely orgasmic pleasure zones. We didn't have to be built this way, yet here we are. It's a gift we should feel free to joyfully accept. (And fear not, if you aren't familiar already, you'll learn about these nerves, organs, and glands in more detail later in this book.)

Whoever or whatever designed the human ass anatomically constructed it for one-way elimination, and some people will point to that fact to support their philosophical or religious belief that the area should be sexually off-limits. Yet breasts exist to provide milk to babies, and unless you follow an ultraconservative religious practice, there's no taboo to deriving pleasure from them. Feet, earlobes, fingertips—none were made explicitly to be sucked, but boy does it make a lot of people happy. What's the difference? If the possibility for pleasure exists within our own bodies, there's no reason we shouldn't enjoy it.

## ASSUMPTION #2: ANAL SEX IS ONLY FOR GAY MEN

Between 2006–2008, nearly half of men between the ages of 15 and 44 surveyed by the Center for Disease Control's National Survey of Family Growth (NSFG) said they'd had anal sex with an opposite sex partner.[1] Fewer than 6 percent of them reported ever having same-sex sexual contact (questions were pre-recorded and answers self-reported via computer). The results from a 2015 anonymous survey of almost one thousand men in the United States, 90 percent of whom identified as straight, were similar—43 percent reported engaging in penetrative anal with someone of the opposite sex.[2] In 2017, sex toy company Healthy & Active released data showing that consumer interest in their prostate massage tools had gone up by 56 percent over the previous five years, particularly among straight men in their mid-40s and older.[3] With anal gaining culturally mainstream acceptance across demographics, and Gen-Z's habit of shattering traditionally rigid gender expectations, it's safe to surmise that the number of straight men who have experimented with or regularly engage in anal with opposite sex partners has gone up since then.

Furthermore, just turn on the TV (or flip back to the last chapter for a sample list of mainstream shows featuring anal discussions or sex scenes) or listen to any podcast that explores people's sexuality, and you'll quickly realize that it's not just men, gay or straight, engaging in or turned on by the idea of anal. Thirty-seven percent of women in the 2015 survey had tried receptive anal sex,[4] and in another survey taken in late 2021 of over one thousand women, with more than 80 percent identifying as heterosexual, 63 percent who'd tried anal sex said they enjoyed it.[5] In a recent Indiana University survey of over 3,000 women, almost half revealed they enjoy variations on anal play, such as what's been called anal surfacing, anal shallowing, and anal pairing.[6] In 2020, the UK-based online sex toy retailer LoveHoney reported that sales for strap-on dildos were up by 200 percent.[7] When women publicly share their thoughts about pegging, in which they penetrate their male sexual partner using a strap-on dildo, they often report feeling uniquely empowered; straight men frequently report they get off on playing a more vulnerable, receptive role during sex.

Then there are trans people, almost a quarter of whom identify as straight[8]—for those still learning, trans is a gender identity, not a sexual orientation—and their sex preferences are as varied as anyone else's, with some preferring to be on top, some preferring to bottom, and some, like sides, preferring neither.[9]

It bears noting that while anal sex has historically been and is predominately associated with gay men, not all gay men want anal sex. Homosexual sex runs on a spectrum just like any other kind of sex, with some people wanting to penetrate or be penetrated, some enjoying both, and some preferring never to engage in anal at all (these might call themselves **sides**). There are individuals who swore off anal sex during the AIDS crisis and never looked back; there are plenty of happy gay couples who are satisfied sticking to oral and mutual masturbation. I'm seeing more and more heterosexual couples bringing anal into their sex lives through pegging. The sooner we decouple "anal" and "gay" and drop the stereotype that one necessarily leads to the other, the sooner we liberate everyone from playing unnecessarily rigid and restrictive roles in life and in the bedroom. In sum, our sexual behaviors and preferences in the bedroom (or wherever) aren't necessarily dictated by our sexuality.

## ASSUMPTION #3: ANAL SEX IS RISKY

Anal sex is as risky as any other type of sex. No more. No less. Vaginal sex without good lubrication can result in painful tears and infections, and any kind of vaginal sex increases a woman's risk of developing a urinary tract infection. Foregoing condoms or regular testing elevates everyone's risk of spreading or contracting STIs, no matter where you enjoy putting a penis. If we're averse to risk, should we avoid working out? After all, you'll strain or even tear muscles if you start weightlifting without warming up, learning good technique, or lifting beyond your capacity. In all of these cases, proper training, preparation, and even mindset is required to minimize injury, pain, and illness. Anal sex is no different. Just as teenage sex is more likely to result in pregnancy or STIs if the couple is uninformed about their bodies and the basics of reproduction, or so ashamed or afraid of judgment they avoid planning or preparing ahead of time, so do the risks of anal trauma, disease, or infection go up when people's ignorance, fear, or shame prevent them from planning ahead and preparing properly. The majority of injuries I treat are a result of bad technique, a lack of sexual education, and poor communication. I don't see many repeat injuries, however. Once my patients understand their anatomy better and practice the techniques, good habits, and sexual self-care that I teach, they don't need me the same way. My in-box is full of messages from people thrilled to announce they're finally having the great sex they always wanted.

If there are elevated risks to anal, it's mostly because of financial and educational barriers to products that encourage safer sex, to preventative medicines (such as anti-HIV pre-exposure prophylaxis, or PrEP, which was insurmountably expensive for people without insurance until generics finally made their way to market in 2021), and to good doctors and healthcare. We have a long way to go to minimize the risks inherent in sex in general, and specifically anal sex, but it's mostly due to lack of access, not a lack of already-existing tools or knowledge.

## ASSUMPTION #4: ANAL SEX IS PAINFUL, MESSY, AND CAUSES INCONTINENCE

Nope, nope, and nope. So much to break down here.

Think back to your first sexual encounter. Was it amazing, or awkward and clumsy? You're lucky if you answered the former, because for most young and inexperienced partners it's usually the latter, and for women and people born with vaginas, it can even be a little painful. That pain is generally short-lived because the vagina is built to receive. It also self-lubricates and expands with arousal, especially as its owner grows their confidence, experience, and ability to express what they like and want. The butt, however, isn't built to receive or self-lubricate, and its muscles can't just pop wide open the minute someone knocks. Getting the ass lubed and ready for action takes time and patience, which means if one or either of the people involved doesn't know what they're doing and doesn't bother to research, the first painful engagement is frequently not the last one. Fear of pain is often what discourages people from trying anal sex in the first place. So let's clear this up right now: Pain during anal sex isn't a given. In fact, anal sex shouldn't be painful at all.

Now, that's not to say there might not be some discomfort in the beginning stages of your exploration until you build your capacity to receive and learn what you like. But through my six-week butt dilation bootcamp, you'll learn the steps to take and tools you'll need to train the skin and muscles of your bottom to stretch and receive comfortably. In addition, this process will help you assess any limitations you may experience and consider if they warrant further testing, evaluation, or procedures to get you where you want to be. How great is it that we live in an era where we have access to care that considers our sexual desires, and in which solutions to sexual problems are readily available? Knowledge gives you the power to become a power bottom if that's what you want to be.

Just as when working out any other muscle, the key is to start small. You'll start with a small tool called a dilator, and from there, as you'll see, with practice, consistency, and patience you'll slowly work up your ability to comfortably take larger sizes. The training is fun! You'll get to set aside a little time two to three days per week to play with your ass, doctor's orders. While it's possible you may see a trace of blood here and there during this process, you shouldn't experience active bleeding, but even if you do, we've got solutions. Eventually this dilation training will become routine, but it should always feel good. Once your practice pays off and you start engaging in anal, remember that in all sexual encounters, no matter what kind, good communication and firm boundaries are crucial to ensuring a good experience for everyone involved.

Now, will anal sex cause you to shit yourself? That's definitely one of people's biggest fears (although there are people in the scat community for whom getting shit on would be a massive turn-on!). Could there be anything more horrifying or humiliating than to poop all over your lover in the middle of doing the deed, or see them recoil in disgust at the sight of a few skid marks on the sheets or streaks on their dicks? Worse, what if they poop on *you*? Humans have built an enormous amount of cultural stigma around poo, most of it channeled into making sure anyone who comes into contact with it feels dirty. Many outside the gay community have used that stigma to paint the sexual behavior of homosexual men as filthy and abnormal. Even within the community, there can be tremendous pressure on bottoms to do whatever it takes to eliminate the smallest trace of fecal matter from the organ responsible for eliminating fecal matter from the body. There can be so little tolerance for imperfection it can send the most willing bottom into a tailspin of stress and anxiety. The ick factor is just that strong.

I can't tell you with absolute certainty that it'll never happen to you, but I can assure you that the risk of poop butting into your playtime is much, much lower than you think it is. As you'll understand when you learn more about anal anatomy in chapter 4, our bodies are literally made so that the space where you'll receive visitors stays clean and inviting as a mansion's antechamber. Interestingly, anal douches, which many of us turn to in order to make extra, extra sure that there is zero chance of any poop anywhere, can actually cause irritation or even increase the probability of losing control of your bowels *in flagrante*. Don't worry, in chapter 7 you're going to learn everything you need to know to safely keep your bum as neat and clean as possible so that you can relax and approach each chance at anal play with confidence.

While few people are completely immune to having some feelings when in the presence of poo—even me, although I see it much less than most people realize because poo isn't stored in the area where I do a lot of my work—rationally, is it really *such* a big deal? Have you ever changed a baby's diaper or cared for an elderly loved one? Too many people have allowed this overhyped myth to deter them from one of life's great pleasures.

Now, anal looseness—the symptoms of which can run from desensitization to gassiness to fecal incontinence—can happen when we overstretch the muscles in the anus, called sphincters, to the point they can't retract properly. Like any muscle, the ones in your butt can get overtaxed if you ask them to do too much too fast after too little warming up. But this isn't a problem I see frequently, and the people who do present with it aren't the ones you might think it would be. While people who enjoy receiving big toys or fists can be at higher risk than others for this type of damage, it's a club that's usually extremely educated, and very good at understanding their limitations and communicating with their partners.

Until now, most of the members of this community have traditionally been older and more experienced bottoms, but as people start experimenting with large toys or inserting fists at earlier ages I am starting to see younger people in their late teens and early twenties complaining of looseness or even rectal prolapse—when the rectum slips outside the anus—because 1) their anal muscles aren't fully developed and strong yet, 2) they don't know what they're doing, or 3) they know the mechanics well enough to experience mutual pleasure, but aren't educated enough to know how to avoid causing injury or long-term damage. So it's possible I'll see more looseness issues in the future. For now, the majority of my patients who suffer looseness have suffered trauma, such as rape; allowed a top to be too forceful and aggressive; or just didn't take things slow enough, whether with a partner or their own toys. But looseness as a consequence of run-of-the-mill anal sex with average dick, in someone who knows to exercise their anal muscles so they stay strong and tight? It just doesn't happen. Even if it did, a loose asshole doesn't mean the end of your sex life, or a future filled with humiliation. There are multiple treatable options from anal exercises and gluteal workouts; pelvic floor therapy, special machines, and nonsurgical tightening; or in more extreme cases, corrective surgery. We'll cover all of that in chapter 5.

You're not going to worry about that, though, because when you're done with this book you'll have learned how to plan, prepare and pace yourself so that your butt can happily handle your next anal encounter and all the ones after that. Too many people have wasted years denying themselves the pleasure of anal because they're so scared of becoming incontinent or loosening to the point they're no longer sexually attractive to their partners. This myth can't be blown up fast enough.

## ASSUMPTION #5: ONLY BOTTOMS NEED ANAL SEX ED; TOPS DON'T BOTTOM; BOTTOMS ARE SUBMISSIVE

When it comes to anal, the more you know about the body in general and the butt in particular, the more pleasure you're going to be able to give *and* receive. That's true whether you consider yourself a top, a bottom, or vers. For the uninitiated, **tops** are people who prefer to penetrate during anal sex, **bottoms** are people who prefer to be penetrated, and versatile (**vers**) refers to people who are comfortable doing both. Though these self-labels are often used with regard to anal sex, they're applicable for all types of sex and all types of sexual partners, same-sex or not. How someone who's into anal sex comes to identify as one, the other, or both can be a product of any number of influences, from the quality of their first sexual encounter, to where they live, to how deeply they've embraced traditionally heteronormative and Western ideals of masculinity and femininity.[10] As we've already mentioned, fear of pain keeps many people from trying anal sex altogether, but that fear can also compel them to identify as tops even when their preference might actually be to bottom. Others who might like to explore different identities find it difficult to buck stereotypes if they don't fit the classic description of a "masculine" or "dominant" bottom, or that of a "feminine" or "submissive" top. The LGBTQ+ world can be just as close-minded as the heteronormative one. It shouldn't be hard to believe that a butch lesbian might not want to be a top. We need to stop typecasting Asian-American men as naturally docile bottoms. It's time we let go of stale rules that say if you take it up the ass then you must be femme, or that a feminine-presenting man can't be an intense top.

Ideally, those of us who get off on anal would all be vers, which would leave us open to the greatest number of dating options and sexual creativity. But that doesn't work for everyone. Some people just prefer to penetrate, others to be penetrated, and that's fine. One thing is for sure, though: the best tops know how to bottom, and vice versa. Knowing firsthand what different positions feel like, what works well and what doesn't, even if you decide that's not really how you roll, can only make you more confident and attentive in bed, and that's always a good thing. Regardless, even if you're a die-hard top who will never choose to bottom, educating yourself as much as possible about the mechanics and dynamics of all aspects of anal sex (say by reading this book) can only improve your game.

As we all know, the problem with labels is that they're unnecessarily limiting. Yet in an age of dating apps demanding that we summarize ourselves and our proclivities in just a few eye-catching words, the pressure to label ourselves has only risen. And that pressure then makes it imperative to match up with people who've adopted labels that we perceive to be compatible to our own, which effectively minimizes the variety of partners and experiences we might otherwise have sought out and enjoyed. This compulsion to lock in our sexual position identity as soon as possible is especially unfortunate for gay and bisexual men, who can typically take over a decade, and even almost as long as two, to definitively self-label.[11] In addition, when used as social signifiers, these labels can perpetuate stereotypes that serve to breed intolerance, limit people's inclination or ability to experiment, and restrict access to the full panoply of identities and representations that should be available to all of us. Who's to say that you couldn't feel like a top in one relationship dynamic, then feel like a bottom in a new relationship with a different partner? Why shouldn't our preferences change as we age and evolve? It's never too late to learn something new. I've had many older patients who were tops in long-term relationships but then lost the ability to keep up an erection as they aged. At some point they might renegotiate their sexual role within their primary relationship, or become single again due to separation or the death of their partner, turn to bottoming, and discover a whole new side to themselves.

Just as there's a spectrum of sexuality, there's a spectrum of control. To paraphrase Walt Whitman, we are large, we contain multitudes. Tops may penetrate, but that doesn't automatically mean they're dominant. Bottoms may be penetrated, and that doesn't automatically make them submissive partners. There are so many ways to identify—for example, service tops, power bottoms, co-tops, vers tops—that I couldn't possibly include them all here. In fact, one of the most important lessons you can take away from this book is that especially during their initial sexual encounters, bottoms should absolutely remain in control and not let themselves be at the mercy of a top. Once you successfully condition your butt for anal play and become more skilled and knowledgeable, then you can of course relinquish control during sex if that's something that turns you on. You can do and be anything you want, whenever you want, so long as you learn how to communicate and listen well, and you're always free to change your mind. We need to let others do the same, which means challenging biases and stereotypes when we see them imposed, and checking ourselves when we're the ones imposing them.

What makes a great lover? It's not treating your partner like a receptacle, or only taking pleasure with no interest in delivering it (unless your partner is into that kind of thing, which is a topic for another day). We're going to go into great detail about all the steps a bottom should take to ensure the best anal sex experience, but that doesn't mean bottoms are entirely responsible for greasing the wheels while tops just get to show up. Great sex starts long before a dick, dildo, fist, or finger gets anywhere close to an actual hole. In fact, great sex doesn't have to be penetrative at all. But when anal penetration is in the cards, there's a lot of things tops can do to make the experience awesome for both parties, from making healthy dietary choices and exercising to remain strong and flexible, to researching the best lubes and bringing a shit ton to the party, to committing to ample foreplay and ensuring your partner is as emotionally and physically relaxed and warmed up as possible. The ingredients for amazing sex—including hookups—are the same as the ingredients for great relationships, among them clear communication, creativity, generosity, spontaneity, patience, and maturity. Also education, which is the only one of those ingredients you can get from a book and not exclusively from direct experience and life lessons. You could be born with the stretchiest ass able to take the biggest dick in the world, but you'll never know it or reach your full potential without educating yourself about the mechanisms of the ass and what it can and can't be asked to do.

## IT'S ALL GOOD

These myths exist to shame us and to frighten us away from indulging in pleasures that other people have decided to judge negatively. Yet there is nothing abnormal or dirty about wanting what you want. You're not sick for fantasizing about coming in through the out-door. Whatever exciting thing you've imagined, someone else has imagined, too; you're unique, but you're not alone. Anal sex is just sex, and as long as it's fully consensual among adults, the pursuit of any form of sexual pleasure is good and healthy and as much a part of a rich, full life as delicious food and restful sleep. My hope is that when you finally put these myths and misinformation behind you once and for all, you'll feel free to open yourself up to all the anal possibilities this book can offer. Speaking of the possibilities, are you even aware of all the things you can do to pleasure your hole? Move on to the next chapter to see what's on the menu, and if you're still unsure, maybe some inspiration to get your imagination going.

## CHAPTER 3

# Explore Your Desires—The Sex Ed You Never Got

In general, even the best school-based sex ed classes—for those lucky enough to get actual medically and scientifically sound information and not a mere admonition to just say no—don't generally encourage much exploration into the vast array of sexual acts, behaviors, and identities that exist in the world. We all come to anal with various levels of experience and exposure, and we don't know what we don't know. I hope you'll use this chapter as a springboard to do that exploration you may have missed out on when you were younger, not just into what's sexually available out in the world, but of yourself. If that sounds like an invitation to masturbate, you should! But what I mean is that I hope you'll indulge in the kind of self-questioning that can bring to light your deepest sexual desires, hopes, and dreams, so you can use this book to help you move closer to them.

For you newcomers, we're going to start with a brief review of some of the different ways people in the anal community like to play. (Actually, all comers should read along; you may learn a thing or two.)

## PENETRATIVE ANAL SEX

For many, the biggest pleasure of anal is penetrating or being penetrated. With what? Most people think anal sex = penis up the butt, but if you're prepared and practiced, sky's the limit! Penises are, of course, pretty popular in the anal community. However, if a top doesn't have a penis, they can use a strap-on to penetrate their partner, an act called **pegging**. Many bottoms enjoy being penetrated with fingers (their own or their partner's); some people like full insertion, while others enjoy **anal shallowing**, in which just an inch or two, maybe to the first knuckle, is inserted. (This is a common bit of play for the anal-curious who aren't ready for full penetration yet.[1]) A lot of people enjoy using specially made anal toys (more on those in chapter 5). And then there are those who get off on receiving fists (**fisting**), large anal-sex toys, even large objects into their rectums.

**TOP TIP:** Fisters (and fistees) if this sounds appealing, it's especially critical that you pay attention to the anal anatomy chapter coming up for your and your partner's enjoyment and safety. Some people who engage in anal imagine there's a "second hole" about 18-20 centimeters inside the body. They do that because they imagine there's a ring of muscles, perhaps another sphincter, that needs to relax and open up in order for them to get something big in there successfully and pleasurably. But when tops have difficulty getting past that spot, it's not because there's a hole that needs to open wider, it's because they can't get past that kink of the rectosigmoid junction. Fruitlessly banging away trying to break through that "hole" is painful and dangerous to bottoms. Fortunately, there are techniques we'll cover later that can help bottoms adjust their body in such a way as to straighten out that kink and more deeply and comfortably take in toys and fists if they want to.

One of the big reasons anal penetration is so pleasurable is that it allows access to some erogenous zones not easily reached any other way. In cisgender males or people assigned male at birth (AMAB), it's the **P-Spot**, which is actually a gland called the **prostate**. Most people report that a prostate orgasm is like a regular orgasm, except SO MUCH BETTER, like a natural whole-body high. Women and people assigned female at birth (AFAB), have an erogenous zone called the anterior fornix, or **A-zone**, which can send shock waves of good feelings into the vaginal and clitoral area when indirectly stimulated from behind, often resulting in a powerful, head-to-toe climax. People say the combination of sensations from all angles can be explosive! You can learn where to find these erogenous zones later in the following chapter, which covers anal anatomy, and when we explore various positions in chapter 8, you'll find I've highlighted which ones are particularly well-suited to reach them.

## OTHER FUN

Penetration isn't the only act that can make assholes happy. The extraordinary sensitivity of the skin around the anus means many people enjoy having that area stroked or rubbed, sometimes called **anal surfacing**. Another mind-blowing act of bum fun is **rimming**, also known as analingus. It's another way to deliver the soft, wet pleasures of oral, but on the anus. For bottoms, it's a doozy of a way to get the anus to relax, open up, and get ready for penetration, though of course anyone can enjoy it if they choose. Some people love being licked like a lollipop, some prefer gentle tongue flicks, and some want to get eaten out like a four-course meal. Other people are turned on when their partners gently brush by or blow warm or cool air on their hole. Most recipients report that whatever is done, the sensations can be breathtaking. We'll talk about good rimming safety precautions in chapter 10.

## GETTING TO KNOW YOU

Ideally, you'd launch into this sexual adventure with a clear understanding of who you are, what you like, and what you're trying to achieve (#analgoals). Not everyone will be quite there yet, though. Maybe you've only recently discovered that your sexual identity is more multifaceted than you ever realized, or maybe you're just beginning to explore your desires. That's totally okay. Even if you're still in the discovery stage, I'll bet you have at least a vague idea of what your preferred anal encounter might look like. After all, something brought you to this book. What have you fantasized about? What turns you on? Who turns you on? What are you curious to learn? What do you find sexy?

I ask not just because it's important to know what you like, but because it actually has a role to play in your overall health and medical care. In my own practice, in addition to obtaining the standard medical history (allergies, previous surgeries, medicines you're currently taking) and social history (drinking, drug and smoking habits), these same questions are what I ask my own patients when I first meet them. Every doctor should ask these types of questions, but unfortunately, they don't. In 2017, my team surveyed over 1,000 American adults (age 18+) of all sexual identities about their doctor-patient relations. Only about a quarter had ever been asked by their physician if sex was painful or pleasurable. Fewer than that had ever been asked what type of sexual activity they engaged in. Only 14 percent were ever asked if they were happy with their current sexual practices, and only a dismal 6 percent had ever been given a chance to talk about things they might like to try if they received proper guidance.[2]

Even if no medical provider has ever asked you questions like these before, you need to know the answers if you want to achieve sexual fulfillment. Go ahead, get to know yourself a little better. Thinking through these issues, even if you can't be definitive yet, and even if those answers change one day, will be the first step in helping you make sure you get everything you need out of this book.

## What is your sexual identity?

"I don't know" or "I don't have one" are totally acceptable answers. Sexual identity refers to how you choose to name your sexuality, which encompasses your gender and sexual orientation.

Your gender identity refers to the cultural and social norms generally attached to the sex you were assigned at birth, either male, female, or intersex (someone with sex characteristics from both sexes, such as genitals, chromosomes, or hormones). Some people's feelings about themselves align perfectly with their external-presenting gender and the gender roles in which they were raised. They would call themselves **cisgender**. Others, even if their gender expression (clothes, hair, etc.) looks like one gender, feel they align more with a different gender (**transgender**), or with both or neither (**nonbinary or agender**). A good tip-off as to whether your practitioner is inclusive will be if the intake form you fill out before meeting the doctor asks you by what pronoun you'd like to be addressed.

Your sexual orientation refers to your sexual attraction to others based on their sexual identities. The most common labels we attach to these types of attractions are straight, lesbian, gay, bisexual, and asexual (or "ace," people who don't feel sexual attraction at all). As in all aspects of sexual and gender identity, they fall on a spectrum, and there are many other types of less well-known identifiers people use to describe themselves. The list is constantly evolving and growing, but for more in-depth exploration of sexual identity, gender, and sexual orientation, I have an extensive list on my website: https://bespokesurgical.com/2022/01/20/glossary-of-lgbtq-terms.

### If you're in a relationship, how do you define it? What does that mean to you?

Every relationship is unique. Some can be romantic but not sexual. Some can be purely sexual. Some are online only, yet sexual. And the participants in these relationships can be any combination of sexual or gender identities and orientations. In addition, the relationships between partners, spouses, fuck buddies, friends with benefits, or any other label can have vastly different dynamics, such as monogamous, open, or polyamorous.

All of these relationships can be complicated. So can traditional heteronormative ones. They can demand a lot from you and your partner(s). So can traditional heteronormative ones. Like all relationships, they experience ups and downs and rollercoaster rides, and work best when everyone involved is transparent and communicative. And while you're working on these relationships, you can't forget to work on the relationship with yourself. It matters, too. People change. Bodies change. Things that made your eyes cross with pleasure once may no longer do it for you, and you get to feel free to admit it. Flourishing in any relationship requires remaining curious, self-aware, and cognizant of your environment. In order to be the best bottom, you have to first be the best bottom to yourself. No one knows better than you how your body works and what feels good. Only then can you give pleasure to and explore your relationships with others.

### How do you engage sexually and what types of sex have you explored?

Be honest. Many people lie to their doctors because they think they're going to be judged or shamed. Doctors who practice inclusive healthcare do what they do because they want to help, and they can't help you if you don't tell them the truth about who you are. I promise, if they've been in the field for more than two minutes, nothing fazes them. There is probably nothing you can say that will shock them. I had a patient once who came to me for treatment who seemed inexplicably down, and I could tell that he wasn't being honest with me when we talked about his sexual proclivities. I finally convinced him that he could tell me anything and I wouldn't judge. His kink was fucking himself with spatulas. That was one I hadn't heard before, but the only thing that really mattered to me was, did he prefer wood or plastic, and did he use the spatula side or the handle? I didn't care what he put up his butt, I just needed to make sure he took appropriate precautions and understood the risks inherent in each of those materials. He liked wood, and he liked the spatula side. He said it created a delicious "pop" each time he pulled it out, and the sensation was incredible. It made me sad to see how embarrassed and ashamed he was of his desires.

Who gets to define what's vanilla, kinky, or obscene? All that matters is that as you move forward toward achieving your sexual promise, you're realistic about what's possible, and get the support you need. However you engage sexually, with yourself or with others, that's your norm, and there's no reason to harbor negative feelings about something that's perfectly normal. So long as it occurs among consenting adults, there is literally nothing wrong, shameful, or embarrassing about anything you do or desire sexually. Nothing.

Your doctors have heard it all. They may have even tried it all. (I can't say I've tried a spatula. But you feel free to go ahead!) If they give you any shit, tell them to call me.

## Do you experience limitations during sexual activity? What about your partner(s)? Is how you engage working for you?

Are you feeling tightness? A spasm? Limitations or restrictions? Are you bleeding? Each of these symptoms can point to a different multifactorial cause. Regardless, though, they're all enough to prevent some people from acting on their sexual desires for anal because it hurts too much, or they start and then quit. Repressing our desires, or pretending we're satisfied with our sex life when in fact we crave something more or different can not only negatively affect our psyche and emotions, it can also ruin sexual partnerships and relationships.

If you aren't happy with the type, frequency, or quality of the sex you're having, or someone you have sex with has told you they aren't, talk to a doctor about it. No problem was ever solved by keeping it a secret, and if you withhold from the person whose job it is to help you, your sexual promise will stagnate. Plus, your story can help your doctor become better at what they do. When I learn about a new kink, like spatulas, it changes how I think about the issues I see later, and keeps me open to new solutions. If you can articulate the answer to this question, you can get help. I promise you it's out there.

## If you're not engaging in it already, are you interested in anal play? What's kept you from trying it? If you tried it and stopped, why?

Frequently, the answer to this one is pain, but it could also be fear, shame, or a situation-specific event that put you off. It could be that you tried to engage and because it didn't go as well as you'd hoped, you wrote it off. It could be that you're a bottom who chooses to top because when you've tried to bottom, it hurt. People come to me resigned to their decisions, unaware that there are solutions to their dilemmas. I just have to know about them before I can solve them. When I ask tops if they would bottom if I could make it pleasurable for them, nine times out of ten, the answer is "Hell, yeah!" If that's you and you're reading this book, you're in the right place.

## If you're already engaging in anal sex, are you a *top* (someone who prefers the penetrative role in anal sex), *bottom* (someone who prefers the receptive role), *vers* (someone who enjoys topping and bottoming)?

As in all things regarding sex, you can be one thing one day and change your mind another, so this answer could change and that's okay. Some people prefer not to assign themselves labels. Some people may have taken on the role of bottom in their current relationship, but would actually like to try topping. And here again, some people take on a label only because until now they didn't think they could have what they actually wanted. Any and all possible answers to this question are acceptable.

> **TOP TIP:** Traditionally, we think of tops as the ones in control. Play the part you want to play, but as you'll see, there are multiple variables that lead to the best sexual experiences for all parties. Learning about bottoms, their anatomy, architecture, muscle function, and skin elasticity—all topics covered in the next chapter—can help you be a better top, too, by helping you avoid discomfort (yours and your partner's), enhancing pleasure (yours and your partner's), and increasing your confidence. And who knows, you may learn enough that you decide you want to go for a ride yourself!

## Do you take recreational drugs or engage in party n' play (PnP), using drugs to enhance your sexual experiences?

It's extremely common for people who engage in anal to use drugs like amyl nitrite, also known as poppers (vasodilators that lower blood pressure and promote muscle and mental relaxation), meth, or other substances to help them relax and thus make anal penetration easier and more pleasurable. The other thing they can do is alter your senses or dull your pain to the point that you can't feel when you're in danger of reaching your limitations, or you've injured yourself. If you're using drugs to enhance your anal sex experiences, fine. But please, learn how to enjoy anal sex *without* drugs first. Go in thinking of the long term—the less time you spend recuperating from an injury you can't even remember sustaining, the more time you get to have good anal sex and make delicious new memories.

## Have you had a sexually transmitted infection (STI) within the last six months to a year? What type? Where was the infection located? Where did symptoms arise (mouth, anus, blood, urine, etc.)? Are you up-to-date on all of your STI vaccines?

The vast majority of the U.S. population is walking around with an STI and doesn't even know it, so don't feel ashamed if the answer is yes. (More importantly, there is no need to feel shame about *any* of your answers.) We're going to talk at length about STIs and how to treat and prevent them in chapter 10.

### When was your most recent STI evaluation? What is your definition of a comprehensive STI evaluation?

How frequently you should be getting tested for STIs depends on multiple factors, including your relationship status and health status. If you're on a pre-exposure prophylaxis (PrEP) like Truvada or Descovy, which are drugs to help lower the risk of getting infected with HIV, you need to get your liver and kidney function checked out regularly. You might be on testosterone or human growth hormone, both of which may stave off the effects of aging in men, such as decreased muscle mass and lowered sex drive. Give your doctor your medical and social history and a complete list of medications you're taking so they can discern the history of your present issue, and know if there's anything in particular to keep an eye on in the future to make sure you stay healthy. The more forthcoming you are, the faster a doctor can diagnose the real problem.

Many people think that testing for STIs is just about giving a blood sample, but comprehensive ones also include oral and anal swabs and urine checks. If your STI tests seem cursory, you're probably not getting the full gamut of care that you need, especially if you're having anal sex, and that goes double if you're not in a monogamous relationship.

### Are you happy? Are your needs—all of them—being met?

It would be wonderful if we could all answer this one with a resounding YES, wouldn't it? It's not greedy to keep seeking total satisfaction and fulfillment even if you can say that for the most part, you're happy. And if you're not, what's missing? This is a complicated question. Take your time with it.

## YOUR ANSWERS WILL EMPOWER YOU

The more you understand about yourself, the easier it will be for you to go after what (and who) you want. It also gives you the power to self-advocate within the healthcare system. You should tell your doctors these details about yourself even if they don't ask you for them. For example, a patient might say, "There are a few things you need to know about me, Doc: I'm a bi male in an open relationship who engages anally. I'm on PrEP and enjoy bareback (condom-free) sex. I get checked for STIs every three months, and I've only been diagnosed once with oral gonorrhea. I'm here because I would really love to be more bottom, but I can't because it hurts too much. Can you help?" Whatever you say, say it proudly. Your doctor should want to hear it!

Your doctors should care about making sure that your sexual health is as robust as your body. This is what inclusive healthcare looks like—doctors who understand the communities they serve and are not only interested in helping their patients solve their problems, but in helping them achieve happiness and fulfillment in all aspects of their lives, including sexually. Whose goals aren't just to diagnose what's hurting, but also to figure out *why* you're hurting, because treatment will differ if your distress was caused by an encounter with a one-time random partner hung like an ox, or by a devoted husband hung like one. Who care to know if you're tearing because you don't use enough lube, or because your ass literally can't stretch enough to handle the size of what you want to take in. And if it doesn't stretch, who will understand that perhaps what you're dealing with isn't a purely physical problem, but maybe a psychological one, too.

I can't count the number of times a patient has come to see me complaining of pain during anal sex after having already visited their primary care doctor, who then referred them to a gastroenterologist, who then referred them to a proctologist, all of whom assured my patient that there was absolutely nothing wrong because anoscopic exams revealed nothing unusual. Their implication is that since they can't see a problem, and the patient only hurts when they're having anal sex, the solution is to simply stop having anal sex. Then I get in there and sure enough there *is* something wrong, and I find it because I know what complications and conditions are common among anal sex practitioners and what to look for, and I'm not squeamish about feeling around for an issue that might not be visible. From there, I put together a treatment plan that will heal the immediate physical problem *and* get my patient back into sexual fighting form.

The second half of that sentence is key. No doctor would ever tell a straight AMAB whose dick hurts during sex or who can't even get it up that the answer is to stop having penetrative sex. They would keep looking for answers because they know that improving that person's sexual well-being is crucial to their well-being as a whole. But that's true for everyone, not just straight people assigned male at birth! The issue of implicit biases in the medical profession—the tendency for doctors to dismiss or minimize their patients' pain when their patients don't share their racial or cultural background, or are women, or are from marginalized groups—is a discussion for another book. Yet it's important to be aware that only half of all U.S. medical schools require that students receive sexual health instruction to graduate. While over 65 percent of medical students and trainees receive a formal sexual health education, only those specializing in urology or OB-GYN say they feel confident addressing their patients' sexual health issues, no matter how much or what form of training they'd received. Almost 21 percent have received no sexual health education during medical school at all.[3] The fact that doctors are ignorant about and often miss issues that are particularly problematic for people who enjoy penetrative anal sex is just one of many examples of how the lack of medical training and physician awareness about specific LGBTQ+ health needs, as well as their patients' sex lives in general, hurts the community.

But that doesn't mean you can't get the healthcare you need. I'm not the only doctor out there who is familiar with and respects the anal community's needs and concerns, and who is committed to helping you feel your sexual best. And there's one out there for you. We're lucky enough to live in an era when even if you reside in an area where a doctor like that isn't easy to find, you can reach out to a physician practicing elsewhere and schedule online telehealth appointments. I diagnose, treat, and follow up with patients based on a combination of anal selfies and sexual history interviews all the time! If you're not getting compassionate, inclusive healthcare, demand it or seek it elsewhere.

Our bodies have biological functions, but they were built for pleasure, too, and pretending that people won't explore and indulge in those pleasures if we don't talk about them is not just unrealistic, it's also dangerous. It's not just unplanned pregnancy rates that are highest in areas and communities that preach abstinence, or where the culture rejects all sexual expression and behavior except what's heteronormative or acceptable for a Hallmark holiday movie; so are STIs,[4] incidents of sexual violence, rates of suicidal thoughts and attempted suicides,[5] and drugs and alcohol use.[6] Many young people who count themselves among a gender or sexual minority rely on the internet and porn to shape their sexual activities and expectations,[7] which means they grow into adults who are generally misinformed and uneducated about how their bodies work or how to safely give and receive pleasure. Yet all sexuality and sexual pleasure matters and deserves to be acknowledged and celebrated. The more we talk about and normalize all forms of consensual sexual activity, the better we can communicate our needs with our partners, avoid getting hurt or sick, and advocate for ourselves and get the medical treatment we need in the event we do.

The other thing that will help us with all that? Knowing as much as possible about how our bodies work so we can safely give and receive pleasure. Now that you've thought a little more about who you are and what turns you on, you're going to learn some basic anal anatomy, and the different types of anal pleasures you can derive from it.

## CHAPTER 4

# Anatomy of an Ass

Being a butt doctor is a lot like being a car mechanic. In both cases, you're focusing on hidden parts most people can't see and don't know much about, fixing them so they look great and function properly. And like most car mechanics, I don't generally get to examine the broken or malfunctioning part until it's become a real pain in the ass for its owner. In my case, the initial damage often occurred years prior, but my patient was too embarrassed to seek help or couldn't find anyone to take their complaints seriously. It's often only luck and dogged persistence that finally brings them across my threshold.

You can avoid being that patient. You're here because you want to have awesome, spontaneous, sexy, fun, complication-free anal sex, right? You can! Check in with yourself. If you've embraced the asshole, so to speak, ditched your needless fears and doubts, and are feeling excited and maybe even a little titillated at the prospect of getting started, you're ready for the next step, which is reading this chapter about anal anatomy. You might be tempted to skip it and get straight to the juicy stuff about lubes and positions and orgasms (oh my!). Don't. You won't be able to successfully act on most of what you'll learn later without this basic education, and you'll wind up having to bring your caboose to a "mechanic" like me. Bottoms who understand their own anatomy are better able to protect themselves from anal injury and illness and have better sex; tops who understand anal anatomy are more skillful tops, plain and simple. If you want to take pleasure in taking or putting stuff up the ass, you first have to know something about its structure, and how all its parts work together when pushing stuff out.

Another reason to pay attention: 99 percent of you are shitting, sitting, eating, and exercising all wrong, which can cause health problems for the general population, not just the anal-intrigued. Starting with this chapter, we're going to fix that.

Unless I specify that certain information is unique to people with prostates or vaginas, or specific to certain members of the LGBTQ+ community, all the advice in this book is relevant to anyone who reads it.

## THE ANUS

When I look at a patient's ass on my examination table, I see a clock. At the center of this clock is a wrinkly little circle, the only externally visible part of the anus. At twelve o'clock sits the tailbone. At six o'clock lie the penis and testicles or the vagina, and the perineum. On the right is three o'clock, and on the left is nine o'clock. No matter what position the patient is in, the numbers of the clock stay fixed. I'll use this numbering system to help you visualize areas and localize issues to be discussed throughout the rest of the book.

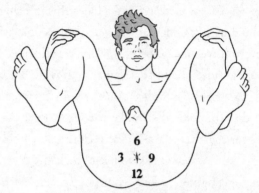

No matter what position you are in,
the numbers of the clock stay fixed.

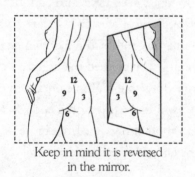

Keep in mind it is reversed
in the mirror.

**TOP TIP:** Hey, fuckers, take a good long look at your own holes.
The more you know about what you're poking down there, the
better you'll understand what your partner needs from you to
successfully enjoy bottoming, and the better the sex is going to
be for both of you.

The anus is what we call the last four-centimeter stretch of the
digestive tract, connecting it to the outside of the body. The part
you can see, the hole, is where your poop comes out, and where a

penis, strap-on, fist, or toy can go in. (Does this information seem obvious? You'd be astounded at the questions people ask me, and I don't want to leave anyone behind.) Think of the anal canal like an accordion, an instrument that can stretch wide but also has to retract and close tightly in order to successfully do what the player wants it to do. The folds that make the circle look puckered are what allows for that accordion-like stretch to take place. You'll see them strategically located at two to five o'clock and seven to eleven o'clock. The folds tighten to keep your poop inside, then relax and open up when it's time to excrete the insoluble and undigested waste products we don't need for health and survival.

That little external hole at which I start a physical examination is actually the tail end of the gastrointestinal tract, which begins in the mouth. You studied the digestive system in biology class, so you know there are multiple organs involved in processing the food we eat into energy for the body, but to keep the discussion focused on all things anal, we're going to review what happens near the end, when we have a bowel movement.

## WHAT HAPPENS WHEN WE POOP

Let's take a trip down the poop chute. After we eat, liquified food descends from the stomach through the small intestine, which absorbs most of the food's nutrients, then passes into the large intestine, also known as the **colon**. There, any remaining nutrients and water are absorbed as the waste travels through the colon in a kind of "M" shape, up the right side of the body through the ascending colon, across the body through the transverse colon, down the left side of the body through the descending colon, and into the **sigmoid colon**. At the other end of the sigmoid colon is the **rectum**. The two are connected by the **rectosigmoid junction**, which is kinked.

Solid feces collects in the sigmoid colon until eventually, as more digested material arrives and builds up behind it to take its place, it passes from the sigmoid colon into the rectum. That kink in the rectosigmoid junction helps control the pace at which the poop moves into position. At this point the feces, now solid, sits right above the anal canal.

There are multiple and overlaying layers of muscles that comprise the anal canal and surrounding area, but for simplicity's sake we're going to concentrate on the ones that control the "accordion" mechanism that allows the anal canal to stretch open to let the poop out, and close shut so we can control where and when we go to the bathroom. There are three sets of circular **sphincter muscles** located near the anus, two external—the superficial and the subcutaneous—and one internal. The internal sphincter, which is part of the anal canal wall, is an involuntary muscle. As the feces moves from the sigmoid colon into the rectum, it triggers motor neurons which tell the internal sphincter to relax. That relaxation is what gives you the sensation of needing to go to the bathroom.

Squeeze your ass right now. Feel that? Those are the two external sphincters. They wrap 360 degrees around the lowest part of the anal canal, and these you can control. When you race to the bathroom the morning after a night of partying or a date with a giant milkshake, they're the muscles you hold tight together even as the involuntary internal sphincter tells you it's time to take a shit, and fast. Your brain receives that message, registers that you're not near a toilet, and sends a message back saying, "Nah, can't yet," along with a direct command to your external sphincters to squeeze and hold. Once you sit down and consciously relax those external sphincters, you excrete your waste into the toilet bowl. Unlike the sigmoid colon, where poop can collect without you

## ASS - NATOMY

| | |
|---|---|
| ① Sigmoid Colon | ⑤ Prostate |
| ② Rectum | ⑥ Uterus |
| ③ Anal Canal | ⑦ Bladder |
| ④ Anal Sphincters | ⑧ Anal Opening |

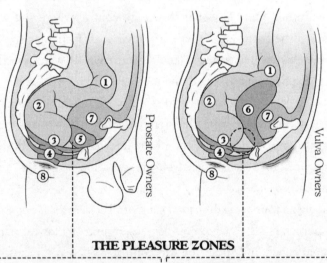

Prostate Owners

Vulva Owners

### THE PLEASURE ZONES

The **P-spot** is a walnut-shaped gland that is present in people assigned male at birth.

The **A-Zone** is an area located on the front wall of the vagina, toward the back (between the cervix and the bladder), in people assigned female at birth.

knowing or thinking about it, once there's poop in your rectum, you're going to feel the urge to let it go. It doesn't hang around in there. As you'll learn in chapter 5, with practice it's possible to gain even greater control over these voluntary and involuntary muscles, which is helpful not only when bottoming but also on those days when you're so constipated it feels like you're giving birth out of your ass.

## ANAL CANAL

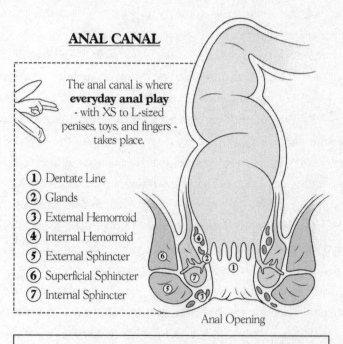

The anal canal is where **everyday anal play** - with XS to L-sized penises, toys, and fingers - takes place.

(1) Dentate Line
(2) Glands
(3) External Hemorroid
(4) Internal Hemorroid
(5) External Sphincter
(6) Superficial Sphincter
(7) Internal Sphincter

Anal Opening

**RECTOSIGMOID JUNCTION**

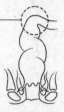

Ever heard of the elusive "**third hole**" (or "second hole" to some)? It's not actually a hole, but rather a bend, located about 16 to 20cm inside. Anything above here is where fisting (and extra long toys) often reach.

Your muscles get a lot of help moving poop out of the body. The ass is incredibly vascular, meaning it has many veins and arteries that provide it with a tremendous supply of blood. More blood means more capacity to fight infection, which is a good thing to have in a conduit made to shuttle bacterial-laden material out of the body, especially one where the skin is thin and prone to tearing. The veins in your butt are called **hemorrhoids**. Everyone has them, and contrary to what most people think, they aren't by definition either a problem or painful.

Located in three columns, one at nine o'clock and two on the right at two o'clock and five o'clock, your hemorrhoids run along the lower rectum and anal canal, particularly near the dentate line—a white "toothy" or serrated-looking seam that marks the transition between the upper part of the anus and the lower part. The dentate line is an important anatomical landmark, essentially connecting the inside of the body to the outside. Above the dentate line, there are no pain receptors; we can feel pleasure, but pain is limited until something hits that kinked rectosigmoid junction, which then puts pressure against the abdominal wall. Below it is where we register sensations of pain or pleasure.

The cells above and below the dentate line differ, too. In the upper part are one type of cells, and in the lower part are a different type, and where they knit together to create a seam is, like all seams, a weak spot—a weak spot in an area that regularly endures a significant amount of pressure as stool is pushed out. Hemorrhoids are one of the body's ways of compensating for that extra pressure. When we register the urge to poop, our muscles relax, and the hemorrhoids fill with blood to create a kind of airbag. The airbag absorbs the extra force our muscles cause when they bear down on the stool coming through the rectum and anus, adding a protective cushioning mechanism to keep our butt from tearing, particularly at that vulnerable dentate line, or seam. Important to note is that these hemorrhoids don't know if you're shitting, sitting, giving birth, doing barbell squats, or receiving anal sex. To your hemorrhoids, these pressures register as the same thing. Your butt in a chair for hours at a time, a baby pushing against the pelvic floor, using poor posture and holding your breath while you lift weights—these are all pressure-inducing acts; so is anal sex, except coming from the opposite direction. Any time pressure is imposed on the anal area, the hemorrhoids respond. They fill up with blood, and once the pressure eases up— we finish shitting, we stand up straight—the blood retreats. At all times, the body works to return to a state of equilibrium.

We run into trouble when the protective mechanism fails. If you're constipated and push too hard and too often, if you sit for prolonged uninterrupted periods of time, or even not for that long but frequently on a not-ergonomic chair or surface (a mistake that has become more common now that so many people often work at least part-time from home), or you use improper weightlifting technique, the valves that control the flow of blood into and out of the vein—the hemorrhoid—can weaken.

Without that proper function, now maybe only 50 percent of the blood will retreat once the pressure eases. So what happens? The skin stretches to accommodate that blood sitting there. As a result, the swelling doesn't go down. You now have a symptomatic hemorrhoid, and an airbag that doesn't work as well as it used to. Continue to impose pressure on the area, and eventually that skin can tear. If this hemorrhoid is located above the

## VOLUNTARY vs. INVOLUNTARY MUSCLES

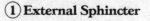

**①External Sphincter**

**②Superficial Sphincter**

The external and superficial sphincters are **voluntary** muscles, which means you have almost complete control over them (try clenching).

**③Internal Sphincter**

However, the internal sphincter is mostly an **involuntary** muscle, which means you can't fully control it.

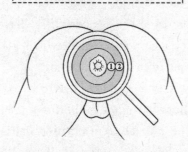

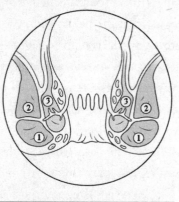

That's why you have to train this muscle to open on command through gradual dilation exercises.

dentate line, in the upper part of the anal canal, it's an internal symptomatic hemorrhoid. You might notice blood if it tears and more pressure to localized inflammation, but you won't feel any pain because, again, there are no pain receptors up there. It's the external symptomatic hemorrhoids, located below the dentate line in the lower third of the anus, that most of us think of when we think "hemorrhoids." Swelling, itching, pain, tightness, and bleeding are all symptoms of external symptomatic hemorrhoids.

In addition to airbags, the dentate line is supported with another layer of protection to prevent it from separating at the seam due to the force of defecation—a column of **anal glands**. Other mammals, like dogs, cats, skunks, and opossums have anal glands, too, but whereas theirs are used for territorial marking, identification, and self-protection, human anal glands only secrete mucous whenever we go to the bathroom. The mucous covers the weak spot at the dentate line, decreases pressure, and allows fecal matter to glide easily over it and out the anus. Yet unlike vaginal arousal fluid or cervical mucous, humans don't usually notice anal mucous unless there is an infection or illness present. In a healthy butt, anal mucous is too viscous (thick) and not enough volume is produced to serve as a good lubricant or leak out of the anus.

But wait, there's more! Evolution was generous enough to introduce yet another structural design to keep us from constantly shitting ourselves. Slung across the body from front to back, pubic bone to coccyx, and side to side across the pelvis are a group of muscles that comprise our **pelvic floor**, which keeps our lower organs in place so they don't spill out. Imagine a woven basket set inside and connected to the hip bones, with openings for the urethra, rectum, and for those who have one, the vagina. The pelvic floor muscles also contribute to our ability to control our bladder and bowels (technically, the external anal sphincter is part of the pelvic floor). It plays a part in our balance and posture, in our ability to bend and move. Finally, it sets the pelvic tilt, the axis along which the rectum and the colon are aligned. When we're sitting or at rest, our pelvic tilt serves to keep the sigmoid colon kinked and, importantly, keep poop stored inside until we're ready to let it out. When enough stool gathers there, or we stand or otherwise straighten the pelvic tilt, the rectum and colon line up, the kink disappears, and the stool is able to easily move out of the sigmoid colon and into the rectum. That straightening is the signal that triggers the internal sphincter to relax so the stool can pass into the anal canal. The change in pelvic tilt is also why we frequently feel the urge to go to the bathroom first thing in the morning when we get out of bed and stand up.

Finally, located all along the anal canal and rectum are **sensory and motor nerves**. Sensory nerves interpret the environment and carry messages from the body to the brain and spinal cord (the central nervous system, or CNS) registering as heat or cold, wetness or dryness, pleasure or pain, and every subtle difference beyond and in between. There are multitudes of sensory nerves located in the distal part of the anal canal, the segment below the dentate line, closest to your anus. That's why we feel so much pain when there's a rash, tear, hemorrhoid, muscle spasm, or other irritation in our bottom. Any injuries, infections, or damage to that area will register as pain, too. There are a lot of nerve endings there to let our brain know that something is wrong.

On the flip side, the concentration of those nerves in the area is what makes it (as well as the pelvic area and the groin) an exquisitely sensitive, powerful erogenous zone. Motor nerves work in the opposite direction, delivering commands from our CNS to our body parts, whether it's an order to tap our toes, lift a finger, or activate our muscles when we're ready to go to the bathroom.

Whew! That was a lot, wasn't it? Who knew there was that much to know about what was tucked up on the other side of that small hole? I promise you that getting a good grip on this information will serve you well as you start training for and then engaging in anal sex. And believe it or not, so will this next lesson. I called it Pooping 101, but I could have called it Everything You Never Really Wanted To Know About Shit, But Will Soon Be Glad You Do.

## POOPING 101

Most of us adopted incorrect pooping technique when we were toddlers. Western parents generally plunk their children on the toilet and make them sit there for long stretches at a time, entertaining them with stories and songs day after day until finally, success! The whole house rejoices! Often, the habit of reading on the toilet stuck. Some of you probably grew up with bookshelves or magazine racks next to the toilet. You might have memories of your parents or even coworkers walking into the bathroom with a newspaper under their arm. Even before smart phones, most of us treated poop time as prime reading time. And that's a problem, because it's not good for you or your anal sex life to spend so much time on the toilet. I won't promise you a sticker if you follow my instructions, but I can tell you that if you do, you'll waste less time on the pot and reduce the chances of developing the complications that can arise from extended sessions on the porcelain throne, namely painful hemorrhoids, swelling, and tears.

Here's what to do: When you feel the urge to go to the bathroom, find a toilet, sit down, wait the thirty seconds to a minute it should take for the poop to come out, gently pat your butt clean and dry, and leave the loo. Don't forget to wash your hands.

It's so simple, yet it doesn't reflect most people's habits. There's no hard and fast rule about how frequently a healthy person should poop; the average number of times the average person defecates can range between one-to-two times per day and three times per week. There is, however, a general medical consensus about how much time a healthy person should spend on the toilet pooping. Once you feel the urge and sit down, it should only take you thirty seconds to a minute to defecate. If it takes you longer than that, don't sit there and try to force it. Remember, every time you put pressure on that area, you risk injury and discomfort. Don't spend thirty minutes on social media or checking emails waiting for the poo to descend. Stand up and walk around. Brush your teeth, drink some water, or do something else. It might take you some time before you once again feel the urge, but when you do, immediately go back to the toilet and try again. If you can only get a portion out and you still feel the urge but nothing's happening, pat—yes *pat*—your heinie clean (with paper, not wet wipes; you'll learn why I'm adamant about this later), stand up, and go do your thing until the urge hits you again.

## TO BIDET OR NOT TO BIDET

Ideally, you should use a bidet or take a post-poop shower to clean your butt after you shit, as it introduces far less friction on that delicate skin than toilet paper. Cheap and easy-to-install bidet attachments are rising in popularity—there are even portable ones!—due to more people recognizing the economic and environmental savings of ditching toilet paper (often people use towels to dry the water off), but they're still not standard in most homes. If you must use toilet paper, buy the cushiest ply you can afford and *pat* your behind, don't wipe.

The stool takes time to move into the right position to come down through the anal canal, which is why you shouldn't try to force a poop when you don't feel the urge. Many people will try to push a poo out in the mornings before they leave for school or work. It's also common for people to use coffee and cigarettes, which increase the production of certain hormones and neurotransmitters that trigger bowel peristalsis (involuntary muscle movement), to encourage their body to move the poop down faster. (This isn't a great idea, as your body can become dependent on these substances to shit, and they diminish the normal movement of the bowel.) Frequently in these instances when things aren't moving as quickly as you'd like them to, it's not that you're constipated; it's just that the stool hasn't moved into the rectum yet. However, when you do feel the urge, you need to respond to your body's message as soon as possible. Every time you hold it in, your stool inches a little way back up, and your rectum reabsorbs some of the water from the stool, drying it out and making it harder to push out when you finally allow yourself to go. Don't hold it. For a lot of you, this will mean getting over your reluctance to use public restrooms. Coffee shops and high-end hotels often offer clean, safe refuge.

Speaking of stools, some people find that resting their feet on a little step stool raises their knees and adjusts their pelvis in such a way to make the pooping process much faster and easier. In one study, 90 percent of participants said they strained less when using a stool, and 71 percent said they had faster bowel movements.[1] Specially made toilet stools are easily found in any home goods store or online. You could also just use a stack of books under each foot. The extent this tactic will work might depend on your height, the height of the toilet, the angle of the bowl, and the type of seat you're using. It's also possible that the stool serves as a placebo, helping you shit using less pressure and with greater speed simply because you think it will. There have been only a limited number of studies to investigate how effective toilet stools really are,[2] but it certainly doesn't hurt to try, and if it works for you, great!

Another way to speed things up is to raise your arms over your head, elongating the torso, which helps you breathe more deeply, thus relaxing the pelvic floor musculature and allowing the stool to release. Achieving that full relaxation is key. In fact, this is one area in which practicing with anal dilators and toys can be extremely useful to someone who isn't interested in exploring anal sex. Using dilators and toys help people get a better understanding of their pelvic floor and what it feels like when it relaxes. That relaxation also encourages deep breathing. All these factors together are why using toys and dilators can frequently elicit a bowel movement. Anyone who struggles with constipation could be well served by experimenting with dilation (instructions in chapter 5) and seeing if the extra attention to relaxation it requires helps relieve the issue.

If none of these tactics speeds up the amount of time it takes for you to poop, the problem may be related to nutrition, diet, ergonomics, water intake, or psychological or neural issues. To relieve constipation, it's preferable to start with oral remedies like stool softeners and gentle laxatives like Miralax and milk of magnesia, and fiber-rich foods and pre- and pro-biotics (more on a poop-friendly nutrition and diet in chapter 6) and follow up with anal remedies like glycerin suppositories and enemas, but all can be done in combination. If you feel like you need to poop and you go more than three to five days with no results—and you've tried all the over-the-counter remedies—call a physician.

Of course, sometimes things speed up too fast and we get diarrhea. We can reach for over-the-counter agents like Pepto-Bismol or Imodium to help us slow our gut down and keep our shit in, but remember that in general, diarrhea is our body's way of getting rid of something it doesn't like. You want to give your system a chance to flush out toxins. Before reaching for medications, drink plenty of water and eat from the BRAT diet—bananas, rice, applesauce, plain toast—for a few days to see if the problem goes away. Most of the time, these bouts don't last long, thank the ass lords, but if either constipation or diarrhea persists more than a few days, call a physician. And more so, if symptoms become really severe and you're really suffering, it's probably wise to go to the emergency room.

A healthy ass is one that you never think about. What's "normal" or "regular" is totally subjective, but in general, the only time our own butts register with us is when they make us uncomfortable, like when our shit's as hard as bricks and tears our anus a little while coming out, or diarrhea makes our skin burn, or we feel itching or swelling, which can happen for any number of reasons. If the only time we think about butts is when we're admiring or lusting after one, that's usually a sign that with proper preparation, our own butts would enjoy some play.

## THE EROGENOUS ZONES

So we've got all these nerves concentrated in the pelvic and anal region that make it feel really good to stimulate and titillate the poop chute. But the anal area has two more hidden treasures we need to discuss. Though neither are located within the anal canal, no conversation about anal sex or anatomy is complete without mentioning two especially sensitive parts of the body that make us feel so amazing, for some they are the whole reason for having anal sex in the first place.

For anyone born with a penis, anal penetration is one of the ways to access the **P-spot**—the **prostate** gland. This walnut-size gland produces ejaculate fluid and then helps propel semen through the urethra and out the penis upon climax. Thanks to its location directly in front of the rectum, it can be stimulated manually through the perineum or through the anal wall during anal intercourse, frequently resulting in a particularly powerful orgasm. Many will swear that a prostate orgasm is infinitely better than the regular kind. They rave about it being a "full body" climax, packed with more "juice" (ejaculate), and contractions. Yet even people who've had the gland removed due to cancer or other common conditions such as an enlarged prostate are still able to experience great pleasure when they take it up the ass.

People born with vaginas are born with an **A-Zone**, an erogenous zone located high up at the end of the clitoris between the cervix and the bladder. Nerve endings connect the vagina to the anterior wall of the rectum, allowing for orgasm to occur with rectal stimulation. The clitoris, too, has two "legs" that stretch back to the anus and connect it to the rectum, allowing for indirect clitoral stimulation through the ass. The A-zone isn't so much a specific spot, like the prostate, but the density of nerves within the butt, as well as the connection of the vagina and the clitoris to the rectum, together create a highly sensitive area that generates incredible sensations when indirectly stimulated through the anus. More than once I've had clients with vaginas who would never have considered anal sex but had to use toys to rehabilitate their holes post-surgery report back that they've discovered a whole world of blissful sensations and orgasms they didn't know were possible.

## WHAT GETS IN THE WAY OF GOOD ANAL SEX

So now you have a better idea of why we're anatomically built to enjoy anal sex. And yet, it has a reputation for being harder than other types of sex, and a lot of people have trouble making it work for them. Why?

**Lack of knowledge and preparation.** This is why I keep repeating myself ad nauseum that you have to understand your anal anatomy if you're going to swim in these waters. They're beautiful and you can have the time of your life, but just as beachgoers need to know a riptide when they see one, you need to know what you're doing and have a healthy respect for the environment and depths you want to explore.

**Inability to relax.** If you've ever had a full-body massage, you know it's almost impossible to reap the benefits and leave feeling restored and rejuvenated if you don't relax while you're on the massage table. Some people just can't do it. Maybe they feel vulnerable taking their clothes off and being touched by a complete stranger, or they can't shut their mind to the stresses in their lives or their to-do lists. Maybe they don't think they deserve the time to themselves or that they've earned this luxury. They're too stressed or carry too much of that baggage we've talked about.

Regardless, for many it can be hard to relax the body without also relaxing the mind. Relaxing is an act of submission that requires a willingness to be vulnerable, whether you're on a massage table, in a yoga studio, or in bed.

**Thin skin.** As the muscles of the anus expand and retract, two things need to happen: 1) the muscles need to relax correctly, and 2) the skin lying over them needs to stretch. If you've ever been painfully constipated, you know what happens when the capacity of the muscle and skin don't align—your skin tears and bleeds because it isn't prepared to stretch as far as the muscle insists it must to get the stool out. One reason for this is that the skin of the anus is quite thin, and even thinner in females and any-one who takes hormones such as estrogen or spironolactone, a hormone therapy that suppresses testosterone. Remember those wrinkled accordion folds we discussed earlier, concentrated at two to five o'clock and seven to eleven o'clock? They accommo-date the muscle and offer support with extra elasticity. The top and bottom of the anus, at twelve o'clock and six o'clock, wasn't built with that support, and so those areas tear more easily, espe-cially when confronted with the pressures of sex. These tears are not only painful, but they also increase your susceptibility to STIs. Fortunately, as you'll see, there are things we can do to strengthen our skin so it can withstand the pressures of sex.

**Tight muscles.** The sphincter muscles, which normally only stretch as wide as your poop, need to expand large enough to accept whatever you're putting in there. You can learn to engage your voluntary motor nerves to help you relax and open your sphincter muscles on demand for a partner, an act colloquially known as **gaping**. Tops love a bottom who's loose enough to fully open and gape for whatever size cock or strap-on comes at them, yet able to tighten up to ensure maximum pleasure for both parties. It's a super impressive skill. Not everyone can do it, but you'll have a shot if you learn how to strengthen and train your muscles and skin through the dilation process, and practice. Just keep reading.

**Not enough lube.** Since the ass doesn't self-lubricate, to protect your anal skin and muscle from the increased friction and heightened pressure of anal sex, you have to provide the lubricant yourself. You won't enjoy anal sex without lubricant. And not just some lubricant, but a shit ton of it. How do I define shit ton? There's literally no such thing as too much, especially when you're first starting out. Buy more than you'll need, and then maybe a little more.

We'll explore different types of lubricant and their properties in chapter 5.

Your ass is built to respond to signaling and pressure to push from the inside out. Anal sex asks it to do the complete opposite, and in reverse order. Yet the muscles and skin, the glands, nerves, and blood vessels were not innately built for that. In particular, to receive from the outside in requires actively training the sphincter muscles to overcome that natural "push" sensation, knowing the right preparatory and relaxation protocols that increase muscle elasticity, and for many, practicing a little mind over matter. Becoming proficient in these skills and techniques will be much easier when you can visualize what's going on inside as you practice.

## CAUTIONARY NOTE

You can do whatever you want to your butt that brings you pleasure, with a few exceptions:

- Never bring anything sharp anywhere near your anus. Keep those fingernails cut short and filed smooth.
- Never insert an unwashed hand or toy into the anus.
- Never insert hands or toys that have been used for anal play into a mouth or vagina without thoroughly washing them first.
- Don't do anything that hurts. (Unless you get off on pain; we all know the rectosigmoid junction isn't the only thing that's kinked.) But even if you like rough play, before experimenting with anal, understand your limitations and learn the protocols for expanding anal capacity safely, so you don't take things too far and cause an injury.

## CONSENT IS SEXY

No type of sex is always on the table, no matter who you are or what kind of play you like. There are a number of reasons why anal might be an option one time but not another. Maybe dinner didn't sit right. Maybe someone's irritable bowel disease or Crohn's or ulcerative colitis is flaring up, which can cause symptoms like bloating, cramps, and diarrhea, not to mention stress and anxiety about managing how and when those symptoms might show up. Maybe the larger-than-expected size of your new partner's dick is intimidating, or despite mutual best efforts, your hole just isn't ready to take on a challenge today. And maybe a partner just doesn't feel like it. All of those are perfectly good reasons to declare, "Not today." In any type of relationship, even the most transactional ones, it's critical that the participants be in tune with their feelings and possible limitations, and feel free to be honest about them. The purpose of this book is to empower you to make decisions. Yes, I can. Yes, I will. Yes, I want. It should also empower you to firmly say, "Not yet," and even, "No." How far you go, what you accept, what you refuse, and what you at first refuse then accept and vice versa is always your call, and yours alone.

Whether you're new to butt play or experienced at it, becoming aware of these fundamentals before taking (or receiving) the plunge can help ensure an optimal experience. Your body is equipped to give you the sexual pleasure and gratification you crave; you just need time and patience to teach it what to do. That starts with knowing how your anatomy works and identifying what you are already capable of and what limitations you're going to have to work through. Regardless, you're in the right place. You want to take it up the ass. I want you to take it up the ass. You now know everything you need to start your first lesson, which begins in the next chapter.

# PART II

# GOING ALL IN

## CHAPTER 5

# Booty Camp—Your Six-Week Dilation Plan

You've seen it, and if you haven't, you've heard or dreamed about it: the movie scene where the couple is getting it on, and then—bam!—in one practiced move they flip to doggy style, the top sinks their giant dick or dildo deep into their partner's ready, round bottom, and everyone is in a state of ecstasy. I hate to break it to you: That scene is pure fantasy. That scene is why the majority of my patients who have difficulty engaging anally, or who get injured, come into my office feeling incompetent or worried that they're defective. Because obviously if they weren't, they'd be taking it up the ass like a pro, right?

That's not how it works. All my patients see in that scene is effortless anal sex. What they didn't see was the bottom doing an "off-screen pre-trial" to make sure their butt was compatible with their co-star's dick.[1] They didn't see the actor as far ahead as the night before prepping, stretching, and warming up their anus so it was ready for penetration when the director yelled, "Action!" They didn't see the actors, who are paid to stay in top physical form, literally exercise their buttholes on the regular to keep their asses ready to receive. They didn't see the awkward poses or repeatedly hear, "Cut!" while everyone repositioned themselves and lubed up—again. And they don't know that not all professionals actually enjoy what they're doing. Good porn is awesome, but it's not real, and it damn sure shouldn't be your model for what good sex looks like.

No matter what, for successful anal sex to happen, a bottom's butt has to dilate. That is, in plain English, it has to open wide. And in order for it to do that without pain or injury, two things must happen: the skin of your ass has to stretch and open while remaining strong, accommodate in a super controlled way, and your three sets of sphincter muscles have to fully relax. Most people need to actively train their muscles and skin to accommodate anything bigger than a good poop. Some bottoms may be naturally stretchier than average, but even they must warm up the region and strengthen their skin to make sure it can withstand the elevated pressures of taking in a dick, toy, or dildo. You'll recall from the anatomy chapter that our bodies have natural protections in place, such as cushiony hemorrhoids and lubricating anal glands, to decrease pressure on the anal canal and make it easy for us to push poop out. Everything we do from now on will be about recreating those protections to decrease pressure on the anal canal and make it easy for us to push something in and pull it out.

This chapter presents step-by-step instructions on how to get your ass into the best receiving shape possible. It's the chapter that brings into play everything you've learned so far about anal sex, and that will ensure you're able to get the most out of the rest of the book. Without absorbing its lessons and practicing its protocol, none of the chapters that follow will serve you as well as they should. It stands as the differentiator between good sex and the best sex. That's true for players new to the anal game, for bottoms who want to improve theirs, for postsurgical patients looking to get back in, for power bottoms who want to reduce their risk of injury, and for people with long and successful track records who'd like to tighten things up a little or add some variety to their routine. There's even information here that can be used for people seeking relief from pelvic floor pain or who suffer from chronic anal ailments who aren't even interested in actual sex.

The exercise plan I'm going to teach you may seem like a lot of work at first, but like many things worth learning, once you know what you're doing it will become a quick routine. And it will only take you six weeks to be ready to rock, and roll, and… well, the rest is up to you. Six weeks is less than an already-fit runner needs to train for their first 5K. You can do this, and you'll be glad you did.

**TOP TIPS:** I can't count how many times I've inserted my camera to conduct a visual evaluation and my patient expressed shock because unlike when their partners try to insert dicks or toys, it didn't hurt. "How did you DO that?" I can do that because I understand anal anatomy, how to prepare my anoscope to ensure smooth, painless insertion, and how to allow each muscle to relax before exerting any kind of pressure inward. The way these bottoms feel as I insert my medical instrument is how it's supposed to feel during sex, except better, of course.

So, Tops, take notes. You could be the person who finally teaches your partners that this doesn't have to hurt. Ever. In many cases, once you are both comfortable with the process, what your partner does with a dilator could be great fun to do *with* them. Furthermore, your good sex will be compromised if you don't give enough consideration to your partner's needs, build, and anatomy. Follow along to learn how you can encourage your partners to relax and open up correctly, and how to troubleshoot when things don't go as easily as they should, so you can all have the best sexual experience possible.

## THREE TYPES OF BOTTOMS

Before helping you become the bottom you've always wanted to be, this dilation program will reveal exactly what kind of bottom you already are. In my office, I frequently send patients to see our pelvic floor therapist, who conducts manometry tests using a special machine that measures anal sensitivity, the muscle strength of the anal sphincters and the pressures of the pelvic floor while simulating the repeated thrusting motions of anoreceptive intercourse. The test is so accurate that without knowing a thing about you or asking any questions about your sex life, our therapist can tell with almost 100 percent accuracy whether your ass will open and respond to the pressures of anal sex easily, with some difficulty some of the time, or with chronic difficulty. (So cool, right? Spread the word.) The results are so consistent and predictive, we've been able to identify three kinds of bottoms:

1. **Anus Maximus**: You can open your hole easily and accommodate whatever girth or length you desire. You enjoy bottoming and actively look forward to your next session

without fear or anxiety. You don't require extensive foreplay or rely on liquid courage or inhibition-loosening drugs to have a satisfying bottoming experience every time. Anal intercourse is easy from beginning to end, orgasm is easily achieved, and sexual self-esteem is high. This category represents about 39 percent of the patients we've tested. The rest of us are jealous as hell.

2. **Anus Mediocris**: Your bottoming success is hit or miss. You always experience some pain in the initial stages of anal sex, which frequently continues through the end. You often have to refrain from sex for a period of time to heal afterward. Some lovemaking sessions go better than others, though, so there's always the hope that the next experience will be a good one. However, because you've suffered pain and even injuries, new bottoming sessions are always approached with apprehension and fear. Successful experiences are often fueled by alcohol and poppers but even then success can be relative. You don't always achieve satisfaction or feel totally fulfilled, and partners aren't always able to reach orgasm through penetration. Sexual self-esteem is mediocre, with frequent feelings of self-doubt, inadequacy, and inferiority. About 52 percent of our test population falls into this category. I know you're like, "Why me?" and it feels like there's no rhyme or reason as to why some days you can offer a splendid sinkhole, and other days you're tight as a closed fist, but there is a reason, and you'll figure out what it is if you keep reading.

3. **Anus Nope-us**: All the recreational drugs and alcohol in the world couldn't get your ass to open up. Despite your desire to bottom, the experience is always extremely difficult, painful, and unsatisfying for you and your partner. Your sexual confidence is in the shitter, and you suspect bottoming is likely a pleasure you'll have to live without. Fortunately, only about 9 percent of our test population identify as this type of bottom. It's a shitty feeling, I know, but don't give up! I've got you. Keep reading.

Do you recognize your own experience in any of these descriptions? In an ideal world, everyone would have access to this manometry test before ever having their first anal experience. By measuring the extent by which the skin and muscle of the anus is able to respond to pressure, you could preemptively learn how easy your forays into anal sex will likely be, and what type and level of preparation would be best for you.

For example, we know that an Anus Maximus will need less foreplay than an Anus Mediocris for a successful experience; an Anus Nope-us might benefit from multiple rounds of physical therapy, incremental dilation, anal Botox injections (they're magic—just wait until I tell you more), or maybe even surgery to enjoy the best results. Unfortunately, most people won't be able to take this test before their first anal sex experience, and many don't have access to this kind of test at all. But knowing these three types of bottoms exist will be important going forward. (And, good news, if you've never tried it, you're about to learn everything you need to know to raise the odds that you're a Maximus from day one.)

## WHAT'S WRONG WITH ME THAT
## I'M NOT A MAXIMUS?

Spoiler alert: Nothing.

People who repeatedly have difficulty with anal sex can struggle with self-doubt and low self-esteem, but there are a whole host of reasons that people struggle to engage in anal, no matter how much they want it! Maybe your butt is only stretching half the distance it needs to comfortably take your partner in (physical limitation). Maybe you have great skin and muscle elasticity, but there's a disconnect between the message your brain is sending to your muscles, and the muscle reflex itself (neural limitation). Or maybe you have a beautifully stretchy ass and great muscle control, but if you're carrying anxiety, internalized homophobia, shame, experiences of sexual trauma or child abuse, cultural conditioning, or you're worried about any of the pervasive myths we covered in chapter 2, the sight of an eager penis or dildo could cause your body to tighten up harder than a boa constrictor at lunch. Functionally you're able to receive, but mentally it's a whole other story.

Whether it's due to physical, neural, or mental limitations, or some combination thereof, what I want you to know is that experiencing unsuccessful attempts to engage in anal sex doesn't mean there's something wrong with you! It just means there's more for you to learn or work through first.

Again, I strongly encourage you to do this work, or all the anatomical understanding in the world won't overcome the factors inhibiting your pleasure and fulfillment. Well, drugs and alcohol might, and up to two-thirds of people who regularly have anal sex use them[2] to decrease their inhibitions and consummate the act. But no one should require muscle relaxants, mood enhancers, and mind-altering substances in order to enjoy sex.

Whether you're new to all this, have already taken a ride or two, or been taking it up the ass for years, identifying in general which type of butt is yours is a good start for the purposes of this chapter and this book.

Okay, enough of the academic stuff. Time for some hands-on learning. Literally.

## BASIC TRAINING: SIX SHORT WEEKS TO A PEACHY HOLE

You know how wellness professionals like trainers and coaches tell you that improving your health isn't a matter of just altering your diet, just increasing your exercise, or just improving your sleep habits, but of making a lifestyle change? That's what great anal sex requires. And like any good lifestyle change, it's helpful to start with a round of boot(y) camp. Just like building biceps or lengthening your hamstrings, it takes time and repetitive practice to train your anal muscles to open or tighten on command, and to get your skin elastic enough to fully accommodate and retract, yet tough enough so as not to tear. Keep in mind that just like the muscles you work out at the gym, if you stop training (or regularly having anal sex), the skin and muscles will revert back to their former state and lose their mobility and flexibility. In addition, successfully achieving on-demand dilation is as much about training your mind, which controls your muscles and the entire mechanism for engaging, as it is about training the body itself.

## IMPORTANT SAFETY REMINDER

Before you try one single suggestion or make any purchases, read this chapter in its entirety. I want you to get a sense of how the exercises progress and what benchmarks you'll be looking for. There will be several keys to your success, but there's only one you need to wrap your head around right this minute: Patience. Learning to dilate at will takes time and training. I've designed my program to be a six-week protocol. Some people may find it takes them a little less time to start engaging easily; some may need a little more. I know you're eager to get to actual cock or strap-on, and I can't blame you, but trust me, rushing the process will only set you back. The comparison to body building works here, too. To build endurance, stamina, and strength, you have to start at lighter weights and lower machine settings appropriate to what you can handle now, then work your way up as you increase your capacity, or you risk tearing the muscle. Same thing goes for anal training. You think a torn hamstring is bad? Try a torn ass.

## WHAT YOU'LL NEED

In addition to patience—so, so much patience—there are a few requirements necessary to achieve successful dilation and ultimately successful anal play and penetration: the right dilators, the right lube, the right environment, and the right mindset.

## Dilators

A dilator is a medical tool specifically designed to help stretch skin and relax muscle. Don't confuse it with a **dildo**, which is a penis-like sex toy used for sexual pleasure, considerably larger than a dilator. A dilator isn't the same thing as a **butt plug**, either. While there are butt plugs that are used sequentially the same way as dilators, they serve different purposes. A butt plug can be left in the ass for quite a length of time. There are people who go to Costco wearing their butt plugs. There are even people getting off in the Costco aisle as their partners make their app-linked butt plugs vibrate from afar! Dilating can be a pleasurable experience, but the purpose of a dilator isn't pure pleasure the way it is for a butt plug. In fact, as you'll see, you don't want to leave a dilator in for any length of time. Butt plugs aren't useful for dilation purposes at all. The neck of the toy is so narrow it can't stretch muscle or strengthen skin like a dilator, and if you're in the early stages of training, you could have trouble removing it. During the pandemic, I had countless patients come in after trying to remove a butt plug they'd left in all day, only to discover the area was so swollen they couldn't get it out. Those who managed to wrench it out were often left with painful hemorrhoids and tears. Save butt plugs for later when you've gotten closer to your anal goals.

Since no one is immune to conditions that can make the body's orifices uncomfortably tight and unresponsive, both vaginal and rectal dilators exist. They're shaped differently, however, to accommodate for their respective organ's musculature. A vaginal dilator is cylindrical, with a rounded top, whereas a rectal dilator is cone shaped from tip to entry portion to engage the skin and all three sphincter muscles so they all reach the same circumference at the same time. While I've known women who used vaginal dilators in their bums with some success, it's because their pelvic floor muscles are much more elastic than that of men, and so the shape of the dilator wasn't as crucial. But in general, the size and conical shape of a rectal dilator stimulates, stretches, strengthens, and relaxes the anal muscles and skin better than anything else, and is therefore preferable.

You'll need three dilators in graduated sizes—small (the insertable length will be about 4.5 inches), medium (the insertable length should be about 5 inches), and large (the insertable length will be about 6 inches). Invest in a dilation kit with multiple ascending sizes. Some come with more than three sizes, but not everyone will even need to use the large size, much less ones bigger than that. The key is to know your goals. If you're hoping to take in a penis and your partner is average size, you may not need to practice past the medium dilator. If your partner is endowed with a larger-than-average penis, however, or you crave a giant dick or strap-on, or even if you're not interested in sex with a penis or penis-like appendage and are here because you've actually got your eye on a special toy or object, you can work with the bigger dilators or something called a cone, which you'll learn more about later in this chapter.

For now, remember: You're taking it sloooooow.

When choosing your dilator, you want to choose one with an initial conical shape and no neck (a thinner section between the base and the insertable part of the dilator). You also want to check the length. Everyone's muscular anatomy is slightly different. One person could see three to four centimeters between their sphincters, while another may have five or six. Not every dilator takes these differences into account, and if you choose a dilator that isn't long enough, you could use it correctly yet still not engage all the muscles. If the neck is too thin, even with the tool fully inserted you'll only dilate a portion of the anal canal, not the whole thing, and the same is true if your dilator isn't shaped appropriately.

When used correctly, a good dilator will work your muscles and skin like a series of sliding glass doors—slowly, sequentially, and uniformly. If your kit moves you from a very small size to a larger size too quickly, your muscle and skin won't be stretched and strengthened thoroughly enough, and you'll be more likely to tear when you switch to the larger size. Finally, a dilator that is weighted and long enough will also work better to stimulate the prostate and A-zone, that erogenous zone unique to people born with vaginas, even if the user isn't sure how to locate them.

The other critical consideration is material. Dilators can be made out of several types of material, each with its own pros and cons. Many people choose ones made of silicone and PVC because they're ubiquitous; most dilators are made of these materials, and they have brand recognition. The price is right, too. The higher the grade of silicone, for example, presumably the better the product, yet even at their highest price point these dilators tend to be less costly than other types. Stainless steel is nonporous and easy to clean, but dilators made of metal are hard to come by and can be extremely expensive. After decades of teaching people to dilate and monitoring people's outcomes, however,

## IDEAL DILATOR SHAPE

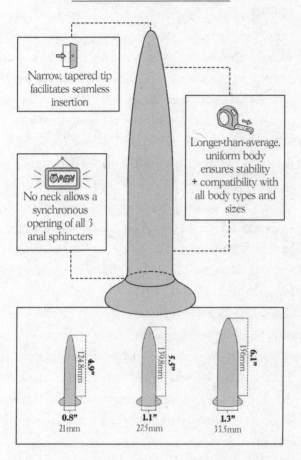

Narrow, tapered tip facilitates seamless insertion

Longer-than-average, uniform body ensures stability + compatibility with all body types and sizes

No neck allows a synchronous opening of all 3 anal sphincters

4.9"
124.8mm

5.5"
139.8mm

6.1"
156mm

0.8"
21mm

1.1"
27.5mm

1.3"
33.5mm

it's clear to me that glass dilators far surpass the others in setting the stage for success.

I know the idea of putting glass in your ass might make you cringe, and they're not the cheapest option, but across the board, glass dilators are superior for reasons of hygiene, durability, safety, efficacy, and pleasure:

1. They're more hygienic than all other options except stainless steel. Glass is nontoxic, nonporous, phthalate-free, hypoallergenic, and won't harbor bacteria. I've had patients return to me with recurring STIs because they've reinfected themselves through unsterilized dilators or anal toys. Because of their nonporous texture, glass dilators are extremely easy to wash and sanitize. They're also odorless, which is not always true of silicone and PVC.

2. They're compatible with all kinds of lube (and, because they're also waterproof, nonporous and compatible with silicone lube, they're perfect for the shower or bath).

3. Thanks to their material, glass dilators are weighted. Their heaviness stimulates the pelvic region more than other materials, and increases their ability to transmit pressure and pleasure.

4. Glass dilators adjust to temperature, allowing you to play with warm or cold sensations against the skin. Just be careful not to make it too cold, which could cause cramping, or too hot, which could burn delicate anal skin.

5. When handled carefully and correctly, glass dilators last longer than other types, and the material doesn't degrade over time.

6. Their unparalleled slippery finish allows for a more seamless, smooth insertion.

7. Once you're ready for anal sex with a partner, there will be no need to switch lubes following your dilation warm-up.

If you decide to use a glass dilator set, you'll find a variety made of tempered, soda-lime, and annealed glass, which are all acceptable materials. Ideally you want to choose a dilator made with borosilicate glass, which is more durable than regular glass, can withstand high temperatures without cracking or melting, and won't leach chemicals or toxins. Dilators made of borosilicate glass are shatterproof. That said, you should inspect your glass dilator for chips, cracks, or fractures before *every* use. If you find any damage at all, stop using it and order a replacement. If you drop a glass dilator on a hard surface, replace it, even if you can't see any obvious damage. Even the smallest abrasion could impart friction or irritation that would spoil your experience and derail your progress.

Full disclosure: Frustrated by the shortcomings of the products on the market, I created my own for Future Method. Made of glass to guarantee proper weight and easy cleaning, each dilator in our kit was designed to ensure roughly five centimeters of insertable, usable length, which along with their diameter makes them appropriate for all variations in an individual's anatomy, including skin, muscle, and the way they interact. You should feel free to purchase the kit you like best from any company you choose; just be aware of their limitations or weaknesses.

## Lube

You can literally never use too much lubricant to reduce injury and increase pleasure. And, no, saliva is not lubricant! Don't make the mistake of thinking that in a pinch, your top could use a little spit on their hand to grease things up back there. It won't work. In fact, saliva actually dries out your skin and makes it less elastic, thus increasing friction, which is the complete opposite effect you want. Moreover, introducing oral flora into the anal canal, rectum, and skin also increases your susceptibility to bacterial, viral, and fungal infections.

As a rule of thumb, you'll want to insert the lubricant into your hole *and* slather copious amounts of it onto anything you put in your butt. Remember, your ass doesn't lubricate itself, so use more than you think you'll need, and then add some more. To hit your deep, hard-to-reach spots, or just to take the guesswork out of how much to use, invest in a lube shooter, an inexpensive, narrow, smooth-tipped syringe that you can fill with your favorite lubricant, or order pre-filled.

A lube shooter is usually about the length of a small cucumber, maybe 5 inches, and can hold about 5–10 milliliters of lube. Fill the barrel of the syringe by removing the plunger and pouring your lube in, or by inserting it into your container of lube and pulling the plunger all the way back until the barrel is full. When you're ready to lube up your anus, hold the shooter in one hand, insert the tip and press the plunger down with your thumb until the barrel is empty. Some lube shooters have a three-ringed plunger that allows you to use more fingers for better control. They can be made of plastic or steel, and can come in multiple colors for those of you who might want to easily switch out different types of lube in the middle of play.

With experimentation and practice, you'll soon learn which type of lube you prefer. Not all are created equal, however, and it's critical to know which of the four types of lube are compatible with tools, toys, and condoms.

### Water-based

Many of the most popular lubricants are water-based. Water-based lubricants are great choices because they're condom-safe and toy-friendly, meaning the lube won't break down the materials from which they're made and is better for safe sex. It's also easy to wash off and doesn't stain.

There are only two real downsides to water-based lubes. One is that it tends to dry out pretty quickly and get sticky. The second is the main ingredient. Most water-based lubricants contain glycerin. Glycerin is the key ingredient that makes a water-based lubricant slick, which is fabulous for providing moisture and frictionless contact. But it also makes the product hyperosmolar. Osmolarity is a fancy word that refers to the way that water molecules travel in and out of a cell. We'll revisit the topic of osmolarity in more detail in a later chapter when we discuss douching solutions, but for now it's enough to know that a hyperosmolar lubricant pulls water out of the cells, causing it to shrink the way a grape becomes a raisin, and die. When enough cells are damaged or die, it can cause changes in the anal microbiome, the colony of bacteria that lives there. Studies show these changes don't negatively affect the efficacy of HIV-prevention medications like PrEP[3] if you're taking them, but they can lead to bacterial, viral, or fungal infections, as well as irritation. To avoid this, and also out of a preference for organic or "all natural" ingredients, some people gravitate toward water-based lubes that don't contain glycerin. Unfortunately, less glycerin means less effective lubrication, no matter what the marketing materials say. Glycerin is what makes water-based lubricants work well.

J-Lube: Originally developed as an obstetrical lubricant in veterinary clinics, this water-based lube has become incredibly popular within the anal community (and with porn stars). When mixed with water, the concentrated powder becomes a gel-like substance that's especially good for larger toys and fisting, not only for its slick qualities but also because you can make gallons of product from one 10-ounce bottle.

### Silicone

Silicone is the superior lubricant in terms of both slickness and endurance because it doesn't evaporate or absorb into the skin. Because it doesn't contain glycerin, there's no risk of causing anal cell changes or altering the microbiome. Like water-based lube, it's safe for use with all types of condoms, as well as glass and metal dilators and, when you're ready, other silicone-friendly toys. It's waterproof, which makes it great for use in the shower, but this also means it can stain, so you'll want to set aside some "play" sheets and towels and pull them out when you're ready for sex, and for cleaning up afterward.

## Oil-based

Another popular option for fans of all-natural ingredients, oil-based lubes have plenty of advantages. Many are made of ultra-hydrating coconut, almond, or Vitamin E oil, or shea butter, and can double as divine, great-smelling massage oils. However, they are NOT compatible with latex condoms (the most effective in preventing STIs), and they can stain sheets and surfaces. While their all-natural labels and marketing may make them seem "healthier" than the alternatives, there are few studies to support that assertion. In fact, no trustworthy studies examining the potential effects of oil-based lubes on the rectum exist at all. Also, oils themselves can be irritants and are frequently made using ingredients that can be problematic for people with nut allergies.[4] If you choose an oil-based lube, do a test patch before using anything internally.

## Hybrid

As you might imagine from the name, hybrid lubes combine many of the benefits of water-based and silicone lubes, but also some of their drawbacks. They're slicker and longer-lasting than water-based lube, and they're easier to clean up than silicone. They're not as slick or long-lasting as silicone lube, however, and while they're easier to clean up, they sometimes do still stain sheets. Because of the glycerin content, there is a risk of altering the anal cells, which can cause changes to the microbiome.

No matter what lube you choose, please, please test the product before you apply it to your butt. I've had a number of patients find they're allergic to even supposedly hypoallergenic products such as silicone. Put a small amount on the inside of your thigh or any location on your body where you can see it, so you can make sure it doesn't cause any irritation or reaction.

Also, avoid warming or cooling lubes. These aren't made for butt play and will irritate your rear end. Don't use desensitizing butt lubes, which contain lidocaine, either. The last thing you want is to be unaware that something is causing you discomfort or pain—being in tune with your body is paramount to preventing injuries. Don't mask the pain or force anything. Instead, follow the six-week protocol and train your ass so you can enjoy pain-free sex and graduate your butt from the Anus Mediocris or Nope-us to Anus Maximus.

## Environment

While there's little more exciting or intimate than exploring our sexuality or new sexual techniques and experiences with a partner, I'm a big proponent of practicing sex alone. What better way to get to know your own body, what you like and don't like, what sends you and what leaves you cold? In particular, anal dilation is best done solo. The whole point is for you to train your ass at your own pace and focus on yourself and your bodily sensations. The mere presence of someone else in the room could alter that focus, and could compromise your ability to listen exclusively to your own body and follow its signals. You want to create an environment for yourself that sets you up for success and allows you to go slow.

You can have the right dilator, but take shortcuts and tear

yourself. You can have the right tools, but not set the stage for success if your partner(s) are pressuring you, or the TV is on, or you've got a chicken in the oven. Make absolutely sure that you feel free of any pressure to rush or perform. Treat this as the ultimate me time. Once you've completed the six-week protocol and learned more about your body, you can invite your partner or partners into your routine. But even then, ask them to observe at first, not participate. You want them to learn what you've learned, and show them how to treat you and your hole right.

Now, some of you aren't going to listen to me, or your partner is going to insist on being involved in your training. If this is you, I implore you to require that your partner educate themselves as thoroughly as you. That means they need to read this book, learn about anal anatomy, and take the advice presented here seriously. That means they allow you to go at your own pace, which needs to be slow, slow, SLOW. I'm always going to prefer you dilate on your own time and alone, but if you choose otherwise, at least make sure you're always safe and that you stay in control of the whole process.

**TOP TIP:** I had a 45-year-old married patient in an open relationship who had fabulous sex with sometimes super well-endowed extramarital partners, but tore every time he bottomed for his husband, who was of average size. I urged the couple to come in together for a few lessons on anatomy and dilation technique, and lo and behold, the husband learned how to properly coax my patient to open up, and their sex dramatically improved. Even if your partner insists they want to practice dilating alone, take the time to educate yourself about good bottoming technique so that when the time comes, you can help and not hurt. It should be said that the best way to educate yourself about dilation is to do it yourself. C'mon, Tops, give it a whirl!

## The Right Mind-set

Remember that this is supposed to be enjoyable! As always happens when you learn anything new from scratch, there will be times when you might get a little frustrated and feel like you're not improving as fast as you'd like, or days where things don't go as easily as you'd hoped. When you're excited about the process and eager to reach your goals, it feels worthwhile to persevere through those types of minor obstacles. But if you're approaching the dilation process as a chore or obligation, you're not in the right headspace, and none of this will feel worth it. Make sure you're doing this for yourself, not because someone else has pressured you or made you feel inadequate or undesirable because anal isn't in your repertoire. Anal should be a gift to yourself, not anyone else.

Shame, embarrassment, negative experiences, and past trauma can take a toll on our psyche and have a negative impact on our ability to relax and feel good about sex, sexual play alone or with a partner, or even about our own bodies. If those negative feelings persist, figuring out where they're coming from or how to resolve them will be key to succeeding with your dilation protocol and anal sex in general. Working with a licensed sex therapist—one who is culturally responsive and LGBTQ+ affirming, if necessary—may help you address your feelings and guide you toward replacing them with feelings of self-worth, self-confidence, and desirability. Yes, you deserve this.

## GETTING STARTED

Okay, so you've picked out a dilator and chosen a lube. You've adjusted your calendar to block off about three to five minutes every other day or so when you can get some good alone time, free of any distractions or obligations. I hope you're excited. Maybe even a little turned on? You should be! While we're still in the preliminary training stage of your anal journey, this is your chance to get to know your body in a way you've probably never been encouraged to before. So long as you go slow—I cannot emphasize enough that you need to approach this booty camp with the tortoise's frame of mind, not the hare's—and follow my instructions, you'll have your butthole stretching and receiving easily and comfortably very soon.

1. Set the scene. I strongly recommend heading to the shower to dilate, armed with a big bottle of silicone lube. It's steamy, it's relaxing, it's mess free, and it will be easy to clean yourself and your dilator afterward. Create a sauna atmosphere. Play your favorite music. This is supposed to be fun!

2. Get into position. The best position for ensuring you get a direct hit when you insert your dilator is to stand upright, or lie on your side, which is essentially the same position as standing upright. If you lie face down or on your back, you'll be more likely to insert it at an uncomfortable angle. Squatting makes your hole tighter and puts too much pressure on your pelvic floor.

3. Sanitize the smallest dilator in your kit with soap and warm water, dry it with a lint-free towel, and cover it in

lube. Use your fingers (clip those nails short!) to coat the external skin of your hole, then gently insert the tip inside so you can also coat the inner rim and external sphincter. You could also use the coated dilator to tease the lube onto these areas like you would with a lip balm; just remember to add more lube to the dilator once you've slathered it all over and into yourself. Fill your lube shooter and use it to insert lube deeper into your rectum and coat the sides of the anal canal. Keep your bottle of lube nearby; you're going to need more, as you'll reapply lube every time you insert the dilator in and out.

4. Insert the dilator into your rectum in an extremely gentle, slow, smooth motion. You won't get very far before you feel resistance. Once you do, stop. Hold the dilator in place for three seconds (*one thousand, two thousand, three thousand*) then slowly remove it. With this initial insertion you're engaging the skin, the rim, and the external sphincters.

5. Repeat. Reapply lubricant to the dilator and apply new lube to the external anal area. Insert the dilator until you feel resistance, hold it for three seconds, then pull the dilator out. Try not to make any jerky movements. Insert, hold, and remove in one smooth, continuous motion. Picture a bullseye as you insert. You don't want to come at your butt with any weird angles. Continue to repeat the motion, applying gentle pressure, but always stopping as soon as you hit resistance, never forcing your way through. As you can see in the illustration above, once your external sphincters stretch comfortably and you're able to insert

## DILATOR INSERT

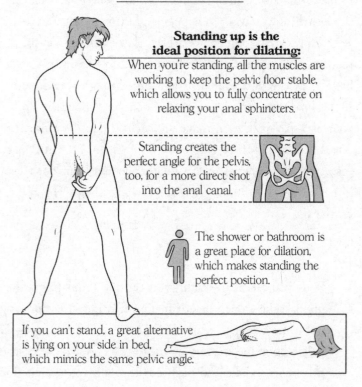

**Standing up is the ideal position for dilating:**
When you're standing, all the muscles are working to keep the pelvic floor stable, which allows you to fully concentrate on relaxing your anal sphincters.

Standing creates the perfect angle for the pelvis, too, for a more direct shot into the anal canal.

The shower or bathroom is a great place for dilation, which makes standing the perfect position.

If you can't stand, a great alternative is lying on your side in bed, which mimics the same pelvic angle.

the dilator a little farther, you'll be engaging the internal sphincter. You'll feel pressure, but the movement should feel easy.

## REMEMBER TO BREATHE!

When faced with newness, uncertainty, or anxiety, our nervous system responds with a fight-or-flight response, which results in tight, shallow breathing to increase our oxygen intake. This also causes our muscles to clench up, which is the last thing you want to happen right this minute. To keep your body, your sphincter muscles, and even your mind as relaxed as possible, try some yoga breathing. Calmly, slowly breathe in through your nose and out through your mouth. Don't hold your breath. Don't scrunch your shoulders up to your ears. You can even make an "ah" sound as you breathe out if that helps. If it's helpful to do it in rhythm with your insertion and removal of the dilator, do that, but don't get hung up on coordinating it all. Whatever helps you relax, do that.

If you feel really tight, you can try simulating a good poop. Take a deep breath in that fills not just your lungs but your abdomen, which should expand, encouraging the pelvic floor and the sphincters to relax. As you work your dilator in, exhale and push out through your pelvic floor like you're trying to poop. Pushing out as the dilator gets pushed in uses the body's normal mechanism for relaxing and helps your body open from the inside out like it's accustomed. The biggest obstruction in anal is the internal sphincter, so the breathing helps it learn to relax. For many people, this entire process of breathing, inserting, and pushing can become almost meditative and ritualistic. It can feel a bit like yoga practice. The better you can breathe and the more fully you can relax, the faster you're going to achieve success.

6. You will probably need to repeat this insertion, removal, and reinsertion four to six times before you're able to insert the dilator past all three muscles and fully into your hole. If you've chosen to use a dilator with a neck, "full insertion" ends *before* the neck. Don't ever push the dilator in past that point. Your ass could clamp down on the narrow end and you could get stuck, then tear as you try to pull it out. Keep your anal anatomy in mind; it will help you understand how far along you are as you feel the dilator sink in farther and farther. Once you finally move beyond the internal sphincter, you'll feel a little bit of a release and a sense of fullness.

7. Once you've fully inserted your dilator, DO NOT take it all the way out. You're now going to pull the dilator back just a few centimeters each time before reinserting it all the way in. At this point you should always feel all three of your anal muscles engaging around the dilator, with uniform pressure on the skin and muscles. If you pull all the way out, your anal muscles will close up and tighten again, and you might reinsert the dilator at an angle and cause an injury. Keeping the dilator fully inserted will keep your anal muscles stretched and relaxed. Keep it gaped!

8. Repeat this movement—only pulling the dilator back a few centimeters at a time, and never all the way out—twelve to fifteen times.

9. After completing your entire twelve to fifteen rep set, remove the dilator completely from your rectum.

10. Repeat the process—lubricating the skin and inner rim of your hole; lube shooting deep into the canal; lubricating

the dilator; gently inserting the dilator; counting three seconds, retracting the dilator, and reinserting it until you can sink it all the way in. Once all your anal muscles are engaged around the dilator, leave it inserted while working it back and forth about twelve to fifteen times.

If you still have doubts or questions about how this should look, or you just happen to be a visual learner, please visit Bespoke Surgical's website for a PG-13 demonstration of the insertion technique: www.bespokesurgical.com.

11. Once you're done, clean your dilator. Rinse it with water or wipe it with a damp paper towel or washcloth to remove any surface debris. Apply mild liquid body soap—scented or unscented, it doesn't matter—and wash well for about three minutes before rinsing with warm water. Once completely clean, place on a sterile towel and air-dry completely before storing in a soft, safe place. If you're using a glass dilator, you can place it in the dishwasher on the disinfectant setting, or hand wash and then boil it for about three minutes in a pot of water.[5]

You'll want to do two to three sets of the entire exercise, from initial lubrication to the twelve to fifteen rounds of constant muscle engagement, two to three times per week. Continue this routine for two weeks (fourteen days) before moving on to the next size of dilator. Each session should only last for about three to five minutes. Give yourself a few days to recover in between each session.

You may feel like you can take larger sizes faster than the time prescribed above. Don't move ahead. You need this time to help make sure you've got excellent control on the ins, the outs, and the thrusts. Your skin needs this time to toughen up, too. If you were to lift weights at the gym and not use gloves, the skin on your hands would quickly become callused. That's a protective mechanism, and that's what we want to encourage in your ass. Every time we dilate, even at the smallest size, we're tricking the skin into getting tougher and tougher. You circumvent that process if you move to larger sizes too quickly.

Oh, but I do give you permission to get off if you feel like it. Just pay attention to how it feels. If you feel any pain at all, remove the dilator before climaxing.

Once you graduate from the small to medium size, you can change things up a bit. Complete your first set with the small size, then do another set or two with the medium size. Always start each session with the smallest size and work your way up to the larger sizes. Doing so not only serves as a warm-up to prevent injury; it also ensures that you're good and lubed before inserting anything sizeable into your hole. Add the large dilator for the final two weeks, starting with the small and medium sizes to warm up, if you feel like you need extra practice or if your partner is above average size.

Week 1: Smallest dilator, Two to three sets/wk (full insertion, twelve to fifteen rounds for muscle engagement)

Week 2: Smallest dilator, two to three sets/wk (full insertion, twelve to fifteen rounds for muscle engagement)

Week 3: Smallest dilator, one set, Medium dilator, two to three sets/wk (full insertion, twelve to fifteen rounds for muscle engagement)

Week 4: Smallest dilator, one set, Medium dilator, two to
three sets/wk (full insertion, twelve to fifteen rounds for
muscle engagement)

Week 5: Smallest dilator, one set, Medium dilator, one
set, Large dilator, two to three sets/wk (full insertion,
twelve to fifteen rounds for muscle engagement)

Week 6: Smallest dilator, one set, Medium dilator, one
set, Large dilator, two to three sets/wk (full insertion,
twelve to fifteen rounds for muscle engagement)

Reading all these steps here may make it seem like this training takes a lot of work. This is like learning to bake your favorite
cookies or maintaining your car. If you've never done it before,
at first you have to follow instructions, and it feels like a lot of
individual steps. But once you've done it a few times and you
understand the logic that takes one step to the next, you don't
need to keep checking the instructions. You pull out your sup-
plies and get into a rhythm, and before you know it, you're done.
Very soon, dilation won't feel like a lot of work. Most people find
it a very sensual part of their daily self-care.

## ADVANCED WORK

As you train with each dilator, take note of how easy or difficult
it is for you. Can you consistently ease the dilator in without discomfort or bleeding? Are some days better than others? How
easy was it to transition from the small toy to the medium-size
one? Can you easily isolate your muscles to gape or contract?

How do you feel during each session? Do you have to work hard to relax? Do you feel like your body is doing what you want it to do? After a few weeks, you should have enough information to be able to put yourself in one of the three anal bottoming categories—Maximus, where penetration is consistently easy and pleasurable; Mediocris, where pleasure and comfort are hit or miss; and Nope-us, where things rarely if ever feel good and they don't improve over time. Should you fall into the latter two categories, troubleshoot by checking to make sure you're following my instructions explicitly:

> You're using the dilator very, very slowly and repeating your exercises twelve to fifteen times over the course of two sets per session.
>
> You're using what feels like excessive amounts of lube, and the right kind. You can't overdo this step.
>
> You're coming to these sessions in a relaxed, eager frame of mind, and using your breathing techniques throughout.

If you're sure you're doing everything according to the protocol and you're still not seeing much progress, make sure to read Part III of this book, which is full of troubleshooting suggestions and remedies. Ultimately, you may need to make an appointment to see a physician with access to the manometry test so you can get to the bottom of the issue. Whether the issue turns out to be physical, mental, neural, or a combination, it's probably fixable; you just need to learn what you're dealing with first.

If, however, you find yourself falling squarely in Maximus

territory, you can consider moving on to some more advanced work. Before you begin, it's important to remember the following precautions:

**Even if you feel like you could do it comfortably, don't hold the dilator in for longer than three seconds per insertion.** The benefit to your bum at this stage isn't in the length of time you hold anything in it, but allowing your hole to experience various pressures and frictions. Over time, pressure stretches skin and opens muscle, whereas friction toughens skin so that it doesn't split, much in the way your gums stop bleeding if you start flossing regularly after letting the habit lapse for a while.

**Even if early on you feel like you can take a bigger size dilator, don't.** You want to build your butt's muscle memory, and make sure you're able to coordinate your breathing, your abdominal and pelvic floor muscles, and your skin and sphincters to all work together. It takes time to get good at that. With practice, some people are eventually even able to use those mechanisms to do what's called "gaping," opening the rectal and anal muscles at will so the ass is ready to receive, essentially turning the ass into a voluntary muscle. It takes technique, and not everyone can achieve that level of mastery, but those who can get there by doing the patient, sometimes tedious work of starting small and taking the time to train their body.

**Pay close attention to what happens when you climax.** If all goes well, you're probably going to get to the point of orgasm while dilating. That's fine—I want you to have fun! However, you may notice some differences in the way you come. If you ejaculate, maybe you can usually shoot your wad all the way across the room, but with the dilator inserted, you find that you cover less distance, or even only dribble. That's because with the dilator in, you can't contract your anal muscles as much you normally do when you come. Some people can't even get hard if they have something inserted in their ass, whether it's a dilator, a dick, or a toy. After training for a while, some people's bodies will adjust, and their erections and ejaculations won't differ that much whether they have something in the ass or not. Regardless, it's harmless, and your erection and climax won't be affected when the dilator isn't in place. Nothing to worry about.

If you happen to feel any pain when you orgasm, try not to climax with the dilator inserted for a few more rounds of practice, then try again once your anus is more thoroughly trained.

Okay, so long as you're careful and keep those precautions in mind, you can consider trying some of these more advanced options:

**Isolation exercises**: It's important to keep the dilator as straight and steady as possible upon insertion, what I refer to as aiming for the bullseye. But as you get more comfortable with your technique and start to feel relaxed, you can start angling the dilator to further train the skin and muscles and encourage them to become more elastic. As you'll recall from the anatomy chapter, the left and right sides of the anus have accordion folds. Once you feel like your dilation is going easily, maybe one week into your training, try doing two normal reps, and then add a third rep of isolation work. After inserting the dilator, very, very gently, pull it a little bit to the left, creating pressure on the skin and muscles on that side of the hole. Remaining at that angle, insert the dilator farther and retract by three to four centimeters, same as you've been doing. After a round of twelve to fifteen, pull the dilator a little bit to the right, on the opposite side of the hole, and repeat the in-and-out motion another twelve to fifteen times. After that, again very, very gently, because the top and bottom parts of the asshole are weaker since they lack those accordion folds, angle the dilator a little upward so that it's pressing against the top of the hole, and insert and retract a few centimeters, twelve to fifteen times. Repeat the process on the bottom side of the hole.

The idea is to put a tiny amount of extra pressure and friction around the entire circumference of your asshole, isolating the skin and muscle on each side. You are welcome to do this with your smallest size dilator if you prefer, as girth isn't really necessary to get the benefits we're going for. It's the weight of the glass and the correctly controlled pressure that's the key to successful isolation. In fact, some people find that by adding this extra work to their routine, they never need to graduate to the medium and large dilators. Just stretching and training that skin and muscle with the small dilator is enough to prepare their ass to take in their partner or toy of choice.

**New Positions**: You'll have noticed that I recommend you start training standing straight up or lying horizontally on your side, but that's probably not how you're going to want to have sex each and every time. As you get close to the end of the six-week training period and feel comfortable and confident with the protocol, you'll want to start trying dilating in different positions to see what works well for you, and what you like and don't like. Over time, see how different positions make you feel from day to day. You need to know as much as possible about what feels good when you're alone so you can try to recreate those sensations when you're with someone else, and avoid the things that don't give you pleasure.

**Build Dilation into Ass Day**: Squats will definitely give you a round, beautiful ass, but they can also tighten up your pelvic floor, which can subsequently lead to tears and painful hemorrhoids. The night or the day after doing your glute exercises, dilate, stretch, and relax your hole to help counteract the pressure on your hole. You're doing the same thing for your ass as you do for your arms when you train biceps one day, and triceps the next day. Each exercise ensures you regularly stretch one muscle and contract the other, and stay in balance.

Once you're comfortable with dilators, you're probably good to go with butt plugs, too. If you have one and feel comfortable using it, you could put it to good use during your exercise routine. Try doing your squats with a small butt plug, the goal being to isolate the glutes and legs from your actual asshole. In theory, you want your dilator to loosen or actually fall out. This will mean that you're contracting and isolating the other muscles, while keeping the hole relaxed. It's not easy and many people can't do it, but if you can figure out how to avoid fully contracting that hole while doing this exercise, you can prevent a number of anal issues.

**Additional tools and toys**: The largest size in your dilating kit is designed to mimic the average penis size, so when dilating, we're training and exercising the first four to five centimeters of the skin and muscle that comprises the anal canal. Beyond that, we enter the rectum, which has a sizeable capacity and is likely the end goal should you be interested in fisting or playing with larger, longer toys. Once you've established full control over those first four-to-five centimeters of muscle and skin and experience no adverse effects from using the largest dilator in your kit (read: no bleeding, no bleeding while going poop, no tearing, no restriction, no swelling, and no pain—only then can you consider experimenting with larger and more lifelike tools and toys if that's what floats your boat, always starting your session with the dilating routine.

If you've been training regularly and use glass dilators easily, but continue to tear during actual anal sex, it's usually limitations in the skin rather than the muscle that impede your progress. When this is the case, I like to recommend silicone cone toys. Unlike the glass dilators, which reach their widest girth near the top and then fall in a straight line to the base; it opens all three muscles as a circumferential unit. The cone shape, however, starts small at the top and continues to expand all the way down. The farther you insert the cone, the wider and wider your muscles and skin are going to stretch. The additional friction provided by silicone increases the skin's elasticity and strength so it can match the receptive capacity of the rectum. Think of your ass skin as pizza dough, and you're stretching out an 8-slice pie to get nine slices out of it. When used in tandem with glass dilators, a silicone cone can truly expand one's bottoming repertoire.

The small cone replicates the girth of an average to above-average dick. For most people who are restricted in taking large toys or dick, it's because the skin isn't stretched or strong enough. The cone is excellent for getting the skin in shape for this. Whether you're using the small, medium, or large sizes, the cylindrical shape of a dilator is the same its entire length, so muscle and skin stretch and strengthen as a unit. A cone's graduated shape with the widest circumference at the base stretches and toughens the

## CONE

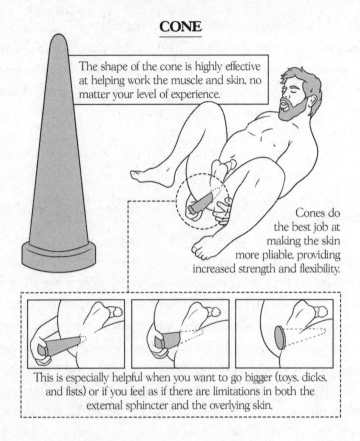

The shape of the cone is highly effective at helping work the muscle and skin, no matter your level of experience.

Cones do the best job at making the skin more pliable, providing increased strength and flexibility.

This is especially helpful when you want to go bigger (toys, dicks, and fists) or if you feel as if there are limitations in both the external sphincter and the overlying skin.

skin at the opening of the anus just a little more than the rest of the skin. And that's good because when a penis, dildo, or toy hits that hole, you want the skin there to be extremely elastic to make entry as easy as possible. Think of cone work as isolation exercises for your asshole skin, and the cone itself as the key to your gate. If your intended partner is huge and thick, you can try using the large size cone, or graduate to a dildo, which a lot of people prefer because it feels more sexual and less clinical.

For people working toward a specific goal, say a particular

strap-on or a partner with a thicker, longer, thinner, or shorter than average penis, there are companies that allow you to design a custom toy. Some kits exist that even allow you to create your own dildos using your or your partner's penis as a mold. These customized tools enable you to simulate the real deal while you practice your anal training exercises.

Regardless of what kind of tool you're using to dilate, the protocol remains the same: start exceedingly slowly and increase the size you use gradually; use a shit ton of lube; stop immediately if you feel *any* pain.

**Contraction exercises**: Ideally, no matter how comfortable you get with anal penetration, you'll use dilators not just for training exercises but during every sex session, whether you're playing by yourself or as part of your foreplay with a partner. The exception might be if you're regularly having sex two or three times per week, which should be enough to keep your muscles and skin in shape. I'd then recommend introducing a new set of exercises designed to counteract the stretch work, just as you do at the gym where you work your muscles in different ways. All you have to do is replace one set of dilation exercises with one set in which you contract your muscles around the smallest dilator you have. The insertion technique remains the same, but instead of working to loosen the muscles around the dilator, you're going to squeeze as hard as you can, pulling in the pelvic floor, like a Kegel exercise. Contract your ass for three to five seconds around the dilator; because it's so small, you're going to really have to work at it. You're not doing this to prevent looseness—very few people need to worry about that—you're improving your muscle memory and control so you can adapt to different dick sizes if necessary.

## WHEN TO STOP

You're going to feel new sensations, and sometimes you might feel some minimal discomfort. However, if at any point you feel pain or start to bleed, stop and try again another day. Even if your dilating sessions go well, pay attention to your body for the next two or three days. Do you notice any bleeding, especially when you defecate? Do you feel any pain, again especially when you take a shit? Microtears will probably occur and might cause some spotting and irritation, but if you see larger streaks or stains of blood, you may have torn or you may have a hemorrhoid. That's good to know. Give yourself some R&R for about three to five days, and maybe soothe your bum with some suppositories or hemorrhoid cream (turn to page 219 in chapter 9 for details), and make sure you can poop comfortably. Once you've healed and complete your next dilating session, pay attention. Do you bleed again? Do you feel pain again? If you notice a pattern, the problem could be your dilating technique—when I say go slowly, I mean it! Alternately, there could be something anatomical going on, like extra-thin skin in anyone affected by estrogen or progesterone. Another cause could be a hemorrhoid or scar tissue that needs to be surgically addressed before you'll be able to train your ass to comfortably take in an actual penis or dildo. If there are no scars or any obvious causes of restriction, you may need a surgeon to strategically cut the hole and then train it to stretch while healing to expand the circumference of the area and allow penetration. Once you're healed, you'll feel delicious!

## EXTRA HELP

If you're confident you're following the dilation steps exactly as outlined here, and you see little improvement over the course of about two months, graduating from small to medium and possibly to large every two to three weeks, with tightness remaining a serious problem, all is not lost. There are several additional things you can do to help coax your hole open:

1. Schedule a visit with an anal physician or therapist who supports all forms of sexual expression and understands your goals. They can offer you an appropriate assessment inside and out, combining the results of a manometry exam, a physical evaluation, and the reports from your attempts to dilate. If they determine the problem is user error, they can show you how to get on track. If they identify a structural issue, they can design a customized dilation protocol and treatment plan suitable to your specific anatomy and needs.

2. Pursue pelvic floor therapy, a type of physical therapy that encourages better control over and relaxation of the pelvic muscles. Following a consultation and assessment by a licensed practitioner, treatment could include postural realignment, manual therapy, biofeedback, or massage.

3. Get Botox for your hole. Yes, Botox, the same product we inject into our faces so we don't look like baked apples as we age. It has proven to be a fucking GAME CHANGER for the anal community. Botox, or botulism toxin, works by paralyzing small muscles, which keeps them from contracting. Inject the right amount of localized Botox

into the friction points of your ass—the internal sphincter muscle, the front and back of your hole (the areas that don't have the helpful accordion folds), and the overlying skin—and guess what? It keeps them from contracting, making it infinitely easier to dilate. The procedure is nearly painless, as the needles used are tiny. Normally, it takes two to three rounds of treatment to get the desired effects, which last three to four months.

I had a patient who'd lost boyfriend after boyfriend because his hole was so tight; not only could he not bottom, but he also couldn't even dilate without pain. Our manometry test revealed that structurally, his muscles had made him a literal tightass, an Anus Nope-us to the nth degree. Baby, he was born this way.

In another era, he would have been shit out of luck, but in this one, he had Botox. It changed his world. The procedure is covered by insurance, but since this patient was self-paying we didn't have to wait the requisite two weeks for authorization. The same day as my patient's manometry test, I injected a total of 100 units of Botox into the sphincter muscles—no anesthesia necessary—and sent him home with instructions to start his dilation bootcamp after five to seven days once the Botox had a chance to take effect. Success! By taking pressure off the muscles and preventing them from constricting, the Botox made it possible for them to stretch just wide enough for my patient to insert the smallest dilator in his kit. Simultaneously, the skin overlaying the muscles stretched, too, so the two could work in unison.

Over time the dilation process encouraged my patient's muscles to relax a little bit more with every session, just like a thick, tight rubber band that loosens up the more you stretch on it. If you were to stretch that rubber band as far as you could the first time you picked it up, it would snap (Ouch!). But if you work on the rubber band slowly, gently, and patiently, over time, that rubber band can double and even triple its capacity to stretch. That's what Botox made possible for this patient and hundreds of others I've treated. And when you can dilate better, you can fuck better.

I can't emphasize enough how incredibly effective anal Botox is, and how easy. It's covered by insurance, it requires no anesthesia, and the procedure takes only two to five minutes from beginning to end. You can resume your normal activities the next day, though you'll be advised to let your anus rest for five to seven days before resuming your dilation training. And no need to worry: It won't make your muscles relax so much you shit yourself. Some people report that initially, they experience a little more gas, but that resolves within a few weeks. You should always poop as soon as you need to go anyway, but you'll want to be especially quick to respond to the urge when you first start getting Botox, because your muscles will be a little more relaxed than you're accustomed to. Until you get used to the new pressure and regain control, I'd advise you to go sooner than later. We don't want you shitting yourself in a meeting at work.

One week to ten days after the Botox kicks in, your doctor should remeasure your manometry pressure to see how effective the procedure was. If you still need help to loosen up, they'll be able to work with you on your dilation if you need a little more support. Should your ass still feel too tight after two to three rounds of Botox treatments and consistent dilation, the problem is probably that your skin is still too restricted. In this case, training with the silicone cone would be appropriate, as the additional friction and pressure will increasingly stretch and strengthen the skin until its elasticity matches the capabilities of the anal muscles.

4. Surgery: Sometimes even when the Botox works well, people decide they don't want to bother with the upkeep of repeated visits every three to four months. And sometimes the structural or anatomical issues identified by an anal physician can't be remedied through exercises and physical therapy. If the muscle is too tight, a surgeon can perform a procedure called a lateral internal sphincterotomy, in which we cut the muscle on one side of the anal canal, which eases the anal pressure and allows the hole to open up more.

Surgery is the only option if there's something restricting or obstructing the anal canal, too, like extra skin, a tear, or a scar. No amount of physical therapy or Botox is going to do you any good until a doctor removes that source of friction or tightness. Not everyone reacts well to hearing this, and I've had patients insist on trying the nonsurgical treatments first just in case they help. Inevitably they don't, and as soon as the patients go through the surgery and realize how fast they're able to progress, even if they still ultimately need to use therapy or Botox to reach their goals, they usually say they wish they'd done it sooner.

In Part III of this book, we'll cover in detail the types of conditions and injuries that can make it hard to bottom, and their possible remedies. But I know some of you will be eager to start the dilating protocol right away, and I want you to know that if it doesn't go perfectly smoothly, you have options. Don't give up!

———

You may have noticed that nowhere in this chapter do I mention douching or dieting as part of your dilation protocol, and you might be wondering why. After all, within the community these two steps are essentially treated as prerequisites to anal play, especially douching, which most online resources dedicated to anal seem to treat as a routine, expected part of prepping for anal penetration. Why?

I don't mention them in this chapter because they're not at all necessary to enjoy clean, mess-free anal sex. In fact, as you've been using your dilators or butt plug, you'll notice that most of the time, everything is coming out clean. Douching can also sometimes make your struggles worse by causing swelling, which only increases tightness. And there's just no legitimate reason to starve yourself before dilating or sex. In fact, as you'll learn, increasing your fiber intake through a better diet and improving your nutrition with certain dietary supplements will actually ensure you a sparkling clean environment for play.

However, I get that the societal pressure is real. So if you're going to douche or restrict certain foods at certain times anyway because it makes you feel better and more confident as you get ready for sex, or even before dilating, there is a safe way to do these things. That's what we're going to talk about next.

## CHAPTER 6

# Cutting the Crap: An Anal-Friendly Diet

One of the biggest worries people have when contemplating anal sex is, *OMG, what if there's poop?!*

Since you've boned up on your anal anatomy, you know a few things that should already be putting your mind and ass at ease. You're aware, for instance, that your poop isn't sitting at the opening of your anus just waiting to turtlehead its way out to say hi. Rather, it's tucked up in the sigmoid colon, where it collects until there's enough to trigger the internal sphincter to open and allow the feces to pass through the rectum and out the body. Unless you and your partner are into fisting and extremely large toys and objects (we'll talk more about that kind of fun later), no one's entering the sigmoid colon during everyday anal sex play. Once your poop passes beyond your anus into the bowl, it should take minimal wiping to get rid of the evidence it was ever there.

However, I frequently have patients that just can't feel clean no matter what they do. Their stools are soft and mushy, taking multiple wipes to clean off. They try to clean themselves by douching—squirting water or other solutions into their rectums—

yet with every rinse, there's more poo flowing out. And then I have patients with irritable bowel disease (IBS) or other conditions whose shits are so messy and unpredictable, they won't even consider anal sex. It can be demoralizing. There are solutions for these individuals, some of which we'll cover later in this chapter. But if you're not one of them, the threat of encountering poo during anal sex is overblown.

That said, while the risk is lower than most people realize, it's not zero, and unfortunately, the stigma associated with poop is so strong that it has led to tremendous pressure on bottoms to do whatever it takes to be squeaky clean. Some people just can't relax if they think there's any chance at all that they or their partner might encounter a skid mark or two. That fear can become a huge psychological limitation, and they often resort to taking extreme (and extremely unhealthy) precautions. Anecdotally, I've heard that some people self-medicate with anti-diarrheal agents like Imodium, cannabinoids like THC and CBD to slow down their gut motility (the speed at which food passes through the digestive system). I've even heard of people trying to control their gut motility by taking tincture of opium, an opioid that can become addictive over time. Primarily, though, many people prepare for anal sex by dramatically limiting the volume and types of food they eat, the thinking being the less food there is to digest, the less poo can be created, and the cleaner their ass will be. Some bottoms literally starve themselves before they intend to have anal sex, which not only has negative physical and mental consequences, but can also become especially problematic for anyone who feels a constant pressure to be ready for sex at a moment's notice.

None of these measures and extreme precautions are necessary, however, when you eat a healthy, anal-friendly diet. That's the kind that produces a swift, smooth, solid bowel movement. A good solid poop is like a Roomba for your rectum, leaving it clean and ready at a moment's notice for whatever fun thing you'd like to put up there. The quality of what comes out of your body starts with the quality of what you put into it. For stress-free, mess-free, spontaneous anal sex, you've gotta think gut before butt.

## WHAT'S YOUR POO TELLING YOU?

How do you know the state of your gut health? The proof is in the poo, whose healthy baseline varies from person to person. One measure is frequency. It's normal to go #2 one to two times per day, and equally normal to go three times per week. What matters is what's been consistently normal *for you*. So if you've regularly gone twice per week your whole life and felt no negative effects, that's fine. The other thing to pay attention to is your poo's consistency. Check our version of the Bristol Stool Scale, a chart that categorizes poo types by color and shape, and what they mean.

Which poo are you? If your poops come out easily—no straining or endless sitting on the pot—and formed—like that of a healthy dog or shaped like a log, congratulations! You really don't have to worry much about poo getting in the way of your sexy time. If they're more like goat turds (#1) or sludge (#6), we can do something about that. Your mission, should you choose to accept it, is to improve your gut health until you drop poos that look like

| BRISTOL STOOL SCALE | | | |
|---|---|---|---|
| Type **1** | | Separate hard lumps | CONSTIPATION |
| Type **2** | | Lumpy and sausage like | |
| Type **3** | | A sausage shape with cracks in the surface | HEALTHY |
| Type **4** | | Like a smooth, soft sausage or snake | |
| Type **5** | | Soft blobs with clear-cut edges | DIARRHEA |
| Type **6** | | Mushy consistency with ragged edges | |
| Type **7** | | Liquid consistency with no solid pieces | |

the one on line #4. That's the kind that allows for a complete and full evacuation that leaves the anal canal and rectum clean and ready for dick, dildos, or toys at a moment's notice.

Most of the time, if your gut health isn't in the best shape it could be, it's because your diet and nutrition isn't the best it could be either. So let's talk about a few simple changes you could make to your eating habits and nutrition that could make it so you never have to worry about poo at all. Adopt these new habits as you start dilation booty camp, and in six weeks your rectum will be ready for visitors to drop in at a moment's notice, no last-minute cleanup necessary.

## HOW TO FIX YOUR SHIT

### Eat More Fiber

According to a five-year study by the CDC, only 7 percent of adults get the USDA-recommended "adequate intake" of 14 grams of fiber per 1,000 calories per day,[1] which translates to the FDA Recommended Daily Value (DV) of 28 grams.[2] If most people aren't getting enough fiber to meet their complete nutritional needs, they're also missing out on one of the necessary keys to good gut health—and clean-sweep poops. Without enough fiber, you increase your risk of a visit from Mr. Hankey. (If you don't get my reference, you poor deprived human, please google *South Park* and "Christmas Poo," or watch the episode titled "Chef's Salty Chocolate Balls." You're welcome.)

Dietary fiber is a type of carbohydrate found exclusively in plants, especially in fresh fruits, vegetables, leafy greens, legumes, whole grains, nuts, and unprocessed bran. Our bodies can't digest fiber, yet it plays an important part in optimizing our nutrition and keeping our bodies running smoothly. There are two types, soluble and insoluble.

Soluble fiber attracts water and dissolves into a gel that promotes several health benefits, such as blocking the absorption of certain types of fat, stabilizing glucose levels, and lowering harmful cholesterol levels. With regard to promoting good poops, the gel slows digestion, which allows the body more time to take in nutrients, and softens stool, making it easy to eliminate. Once the soluble fiber hits the large intestine, a.k.a. the colon, it ferments and becomes food for the gut bacteria residing there, which turn it into energy. Foods high in soluble fiber include black beans, lentils, oats, edamame, Brussels sprouts, chia seeds, avocados, and fruits such as citrus (mostly in the peels), pears, apples, strawberries, and, of course, peaches.

Insoluble fiber remains intact as it moves through your system, absorbing water and adding bulk to your stool. Bulky stool is soft stool that comes out easily and leaves you feeling clean without having to wipe yourself repeatedly. It has other benefits, too. That bulk helps "scrub" the sides of the intestines, which helps keep it clear of toxins and other waste, thus possibly reducing the risk of colon cancer[3]. It helps stimulate peristalsis, the wave-like muscle contractions that push the stool through the colon to the rectum and out the anus, preventing not just constipation, hemorrhoids,[4] and fissures. It can also decrease the risk of diverticulitis flare-ups[5], which is when little pockets in the lining of the colon become inflamed or infected, which can be painful. Foods especially high in insoluble fiber are the kind we're told to eat when we need more "roughage," like whole wheat, cauliflower, nuts, seeds, dark leafy vegetables, beans, unpeeled potatoes, and celery.

Most fiber-rich foods contain a combination of both soluble and insoluble fiber in varying amounts. It's also worth noting that canned and frozen fruits and vegetables are just as good sources of fiber as raw, steamed, or roasted.[6] The important thing is to make a conscious effort to increase the number of servings and the variety of sources in your diet as much as you can.

With so many benefits to eating fiber, why do so many of us get an inadequate amount? One reason is our Western diet, which emphasizes processed and refined carbohydrates that have had the fiber removed—white breads, pastas, and chips, for example. When our tastes have been shaped by foods high in fat, salt, and sugar, more nutritious options like whole grains, brown breads, and unadulterated fruits and vegetables can be tough to swallow. They're delicious when prepared properly, but for people who have less time or less inclination to cook, they can feel like more work than they're worth. In some low-income communities, it can be hard to find a large selection of these types of foods, or even a supermarket. Canned and frozen fruits and vegetables have a longer shelf life and take less time to prepare than fresh, but they're also more expensive; whole grains and legumes, too, are usually more expensive and take more time to cook in their raw or nutritionally whole versions than when processed or turned into instant-cook products. These are legitimate logistical and financial challenges to improving the nutritional values in your diet. However, you can at least increase your fiber intake without making radical, expensive changes. For example, you might:

1. Shake up your breakfast routine with a smoothie made with a base of apple, banana, or pear.
2. Replace your morning bagel or toast with a whole-grain version. Add even more fiber by sometimes replacing the cream cheese with avocado or nut butter.
3. Throw steel-cut or rolled oats (not instant oatmeal, which has had most of the fiber stripped out) with milk or water

in a crockpot set to low at night and wake up to a ready-made breakfast. Top it with some nuts and berries for an extra fiber boost.

4. Add a side salad to your lunches. Any kind will do, just be careful not to add too much cheese and dressing. The pre-packaged ones you can find at most supermarkets make life easy (the shredded kale-and-brussels sprouts variety is particularly nutrient dense).

5. Add extra beans and legumes to a favorite soup or stew.

As you can see, this shit doesn't have to be hard! My favorite fiber booster is Chia seeds. They're almost pure soluble fiber and highly versatile. Add a tablespoon to smoothies, soups, stews, or baked goods like muffins, where the seeds will act as a thickener but not affect the taste. When soaked, they become gummy, and many people enjoy them sweetened and served as a pudding-like dessert. You can also sprinkle them raw on pretty much anything for added texture.

Don't overdo things—too much soluble fiber can make you constipated; too much insoluble fiber can give you diarrhea. Too much of any kind of fiber, and you could wind up with a bad case of gas. Treat your digestive system delicately by starting small and giving your body time to adjust. For example, introduce each element of your new fiber-rich diet—a cup of fruit, a spoonful of chia, salad with lunch or dinner—one at a time over the course of a few days and see how your body reacts. If you're a meat-and-potatoes kind of person and not accustomed to loading up on fiber, adding an avalanche of fruits and vegetables to your diet overnight will set you up for a painful case of the runs. Balance that fiber out by substituting the high-fat red meat on your plate with portions of lean protein like chicken breast, pork tenderloin, or turkey. As always, go slow. As you start adding more fiber to your diet and making these changes, you should notice that your bowels are evacuating more frequently, and your stools are softer (though not mushy), larger, and getting closer to looking like the example on the fourth line of the Bristol stool chart. That's the one that will leave your ass anal-sex ready.

## FIBER ON THE GO

It's almost impossible to cook from scratch all the time, and not everyone enjoys it. If you don't want to rely exclusively on raw fruits and veggies, you'll need to learn to read the nutritional labels on packaged foods to see what items have good sources of fiber, and which are just marketed to make you think they do. As you now know, the FDA's Recommended Daily Value (DV) is 28g of fiber. When you read a nutrition label, you'll want to look for another number, the Percent Daily Value (%DV). That's the number indicating what percentage of your total DV can be found in a single serving of the product. According to the website of the Food and Drug Administration (FDA):

"5% DV or less of a nutrient per serving is considered low. 20% DV or more of a nutrient per serving is considered high."[7]

Everybody's needs are different. Some people will need a little more fiber to achieve bottoming-friendly shits, some will need a little less. Just try to add more products to your basket or online order that have a fiber content ranging somewhere in between these ranges, and you'll be doing great.

## Drink More Water

Our bodies are made up almost entirely of water, and water plays a huge role in determining the quality of our gut health, poo size and texture, and gut motility (how fast food and water move through your digestive tract). How many servings per day you actually require depends on many factors, including your weight, your level of physical activity, or whether you live in a humid or dry environment. It also depends on your diet. You, anal engager, are trying to eat more fiber to improve the quality of your poops, and that means you will have to drink even more water. Remember that insoluble fiber draws water into poop to create bulk and keep it soft and propulsive so that it can move through you and be expelled faster. If you don't take in enough water, your body will use what water it does get to support the rest of your functions, and there won't be anything left for the stool, leaving you straining to pass a rock-hard shit that could possibly tear your anus, or at the very least leave you feeling bloated and uncomfortable. None of that makes for a happy, sex-ready asshole.

The general recommendation for fluid intake per day is about 15.5 cups for men, and 11.5 cups for women.[8] One easy way to know whether you're getting enough is to check the color of your urine. A well-hydrated body expels light yellow urine; darker colored urine means you need to ingest more water.[9] Keep filled cups and bottles near you so you can take regular sips (if you're drinking when you're thirsty, you're already dehydrated; a water bottle printed with time markers is a great way to help you remember to keep drinking through the day. Your body will also absorb water from the food you eat, so you can boost your water intake by eating lots of water-rich fruits and vegetables like melons, strawberries, cucumbers, lettuce, celery, zucchini and yellow squash, bell peppers, and spinach.[10]

## Fiber Supplements

If you're one of those people who just aren't that interested in cooking or thinking more about what they eat, or you don't see a positive change in your bowel habits after a few days of adding more fiber to your diet, supplements are an easy addition you can make to your daily routine to boost your fiber intake so you're more likely to produce bottoming-friendly BMs. Among the common types of fiber used in these types of supplements are psyllium husk and acacia, both soluble fibers, the kind that turns to gel once it gets into your system. Both can be found in all kinds of packaged food products, but in the form of powders, pills, and capsules they work well to bulk up your poo, and help soften it by pulling water into your GI tract. In addition, both promote a sense of satiety and fullness, which not only helps with weight control, but also means fewer bowel movements in general.[11]

A few cautionary notes about fiber supplements:

Some can interfere with medications, so speak to your doctor before starting a fiber supplement regimen.

Hydrate, hydrate, hydrate! Anyone taking fiber supplements must make it a priority to follow the instructions on the supplement package, which generally include consuming large glasses of water with each dose. If you eat more fiber, or take a fiber supplement, and don't follow up with plentiful amounts of water, you're likely to become constipated. Many of us love rock-hard dick; rock-hard poop, not so much.

Start slow. Some fiber supplements will have you take four to six pills per day, but you may not need that many to see beneficial results, and taking more than necessary could cause constipation. If you're going to add fiber from whole-food sources into your diet, do that first and see what happens. Then give it a month to see if it's working before changing anything in your routine. That way, you'll know what benefits you've gained from adding fiber to your diet, and what can be attributed to the supplement once you start taking it. If the supplement calls for twice daily doses, consider starting with just one dose and seeing how that affects your system. It may be all you need.

Timing counts. I like to recommend taking fiber supplements at night before bed, primarily because it decreases the risk of the supplements interfering with any medications you may take earlier in the day. Since we're not moving around much, it's also when our bodies are working on peak absorption. We can't drink water to replenish what we expend while we're sleeping, so our body pulls excess water from wherever it can find it, namely the tissue in our legs and feet, which is good for the bowel. Taking the supplements at night will prime you for your morning poop reflex, which you'll recall from the anatomy chapter is initiated when you get out of bed and stand up, thus changing your pelvic angle.

Keep in mind that fiber supplements affect every body differently, with some people seeing immediate benefits, and others finding that it sets off an inflammatory response or other negative effects. One thing that does seem to be consistent, however, is that they all alter the microbiome,[12] the colony of trillions of bacteria that primarily live in our gut, though they're present in and on other parts of the body. The composition of your gut microbiome affects the efficacy of your digestion and the consistency of your stool.[13] The more robust and diverse the composition of your microbiome, the better your gut health, and anything that promotes optimal gut health makes for better anal sex.

## Prebiotics and Probiotics

There are two ways we can help our bodies stay in balance and replenish our microbiome. The first way is introducing more bacteria to your system, much like restocking a koi pond. Many foods already contain the bacteria our bodies need, and when we consume them, they add to the general population of our microbiome. Maybe you've heard that fermented foods like sauerkraut, kimchi, kombucha, yogurt, and even sourdough bread are good for the gut. That's because the fermentation process that creates them supports the production of the kind of live bacteria that's good for us, called probiotics. When we eat these products, more of those probiotics make their way into the gut and help support the population already there. If you don't like the kinds of foods that are rich in probiotics, however, you're in luck, as you can also take probiotics via a daily pill. Bifidobacterium and Lactobacillus are two of the most common strains.

Now, like all living things, the bacteria that resides in our gut has to eat or it will die. What it eats are called prebiotics, and all prebiotics are derived from dietary fiber. Yes, we're talking about fiber again! That means acacia and psyllium husk—some of the most effective fiber supplements—may act as prebiotics.[14] While researchers still aren't sure how prebiotics work,[15] research does indicate that they ease constipation and bloating,[16] a common symptom for people with low-fiber diets. Prebiotics, like probiotics, are naturally found in many of the foods we consume, but to guarantee that you get enough, these, too, are available in a daily supplement.

For the best of both pre- and probiotic worlds, there are synbiotics, which are specially formulated combinations of the two delivered in one supplement. Probiotics have to survive a pretty inhospitable acidic environment as they make their way through the body. Scientists have found that supporting probiotics with properly matched prebiotics helps protect the good bacteria so that it can make its way past the upper gastrointestinal tract and into the large intestine and colon.[17] This is great, as improved gut health is always beneficial. Unfortunately, most synbiotic supplements still aren't anal specific; they're not designed to get past the colon (large intestine) to the rectum and anal area. I see this as a problem for anal engagers. For example, anal sex can promote a buildup of a bacteria called Prevotella, which can overwhelm the anal microbiome and increase the risk of STIs and injury[18], and we've found that pre- and probiotics replenish the good bacteria so the Prevotella can't repopulate. Few if any traditional pre- or probiotics or synbiotics would be able to deliver that lactobacillus to the affected area. Ultimately, frustrated by the lack of reliable supplements that could repopulate the booty biome, I created one for Future Method.

It's not just what you eat that alters your microbiome. Sex can do it, too. Think about all that lubing and sucking and fucking and touching and penetrating good sex entails. Sexually active people swap a lot of microbes. Like, a lot. And yet keeping the good and bad bacteria of the microbiome in a state of homeostasis is essential to overall health, as well as anal health because one of the other places besides the gut where the microbiome exists is the butt. When that booty biome is altered, we may see higher rates of HIV and other STIs[19], which can make people more vulnerable to other anal injuries as well.

Anyone on the receiving end of anal sex should make it a point to take pre- and probiotics for their gut health. Due to the way we play and have sex, we consume more types of bacteria that can alter our microbiomes. Without controlling for this, the community is more susceptible to infections like *H. pylori*—which can infect the stomach—and Irritable Bowel Syndrome (IBS) and Small Intestine Bacterial Overgrowth (SIBO), which are especially prevalent in males who receive anal sex. Symptoms can include intense digestive tract discomfort in the form of gas and frequent constipation, diarrhea, and bloating, and it's often mistaken for IBS, especially by doctors who don't think to ask their patients if they engage in anal intercourse. In addition, dysbiosis—an imbalanced gut microbiome—can lead to inflammatory bowel diseases (IBD) like Crohn's and ulcerative colitis. In fact, homosexual men are twice as likely to be diagnosed with IBD than heterosexual men, even when both engage in high-risk sexual activity.[20] See the end of this chapter for advice on what to do if you're afflicted with any of these conditions.

## Control Your Gut Transit Time

Did you know that what you eat today doesn't necessarily get pooped out tomorrow? Depending on what you eat, it can take anywhere from twenty-four hours to as long as *five days* for the food you eat to get fully digested and make its way out of the body.[21] For people into anal, that unpredictability can be nerve-wracking.

Your gut transit time refers to the amount of time it takes for the food you eat to make its way from your mouth to the toilet bowl. It's another measure you can use to gauge how what you eat is affecting your gut health and your bowel movements, and help you make good decisions when you're considering or planning anal sex. Some people who love anal like to be aware of their digestive patterns and rhythms so they can arrange anal sex when they're least likely to have poop in their system, thus reducing the risk of streaks or embarrassing accidents. An easy way to get a baseline knowledge of how long your body takes to digest its food is to eat something indigestible, then track how long it takes before you see that food in your stool. A doctor might have you swallow a special pill or dye, but you can accomplish the same thing by swallowing a few cooked corn kernels at home. Our bodies can't digest the outer husk of corn kernels, so they come out studded through your stool in almost exactly the same form as they went in, making them easy to spot in the toilet bowel.

We've already mentioned several inadvisable ways people try to alter their transit time so they feel ready and comfortable for sex. Some people will stop eating. Others take medications like Imodium or Pepto Bismol, or narcotics like tincture of opium, all of which can burn out the muscle motion (peristalsis) of your intestines and cause chronic constipation. Adopting an anal-friendly diet and good nutrition is a much gentler, more natural, and equally effective way to achieve the same end. Of course you should start by keeping track of how your body reacts to certain foods; if greasy pizza runs through you, that's probably something you'll want to keep in mind the next time it looks like sex might be in the cards. But you can also make sustainable, long-term changes. If your poos are mushy and soft and rush out of you just hours after you eat, or are too hard and take days to pass, try increasing your fiber intake and hydration and start taking pre- and probiotics. See how that affects your transit time and poo consistency. Are you starting to regularly see poos that match the ideal example on the Bristol stool chart? Not yet? Try adding some fiber supplements. Take it slow and easy, and adjust until you can predict with close accuracy when you'll be due for a bowel movement. Once you've got a rhythm down and your stools are soft, firm, and easy to pass, you should be able to plan poop-free sex accordingly without having to stress about mess—or going hungry!

If making these changes to your diet doesn't have any effect over time, you should get evaluated by your doctor or even a gastroenterologist. You'll want to get tested to make sure you haven't contracted a parasite or other ailment that can produce these symptoms.

## HOW TO AVOID DIARRHEA

Sometimes we don't mean to alter our normal, predictable transit time, but then we get hit with a virus, infection, intolerance or allergy, or we take a new medication like an antibiotic, and we get diarrhea. Certain foods, too, are more likely than others to cause your body to react in unpleasant ways. If you believe anal sex is in your future and you want to do what you can to make sure that a) when you poop there are no stragglers left behind, and b) you're not hit with the urge to purge at an indiscreet moment, be conscious of the amount you consume of the following:

**Spicy foods.** Our mouth burns when we eat spicy food because the capsaicin triggers pain receptors that tell our brains that our bodies are burning from the inside. Once we swallow, the capsaicin sends the same message to the pain sensors in the digestive tract. In some people, as the intestines get irritated, they move to get rid of the pain instigator, which leads the gut to speed the food along[22]—faster than the stool can absorb the water in the gut. Too-fast transit time = watery stool = diarrhea.

**Fat.** Fat-laden, greasy foods taste great going down, but even in moderate amounts they can easily overwhelm the digestive system and trigger a dash to the bathroom. Additionally, a lot of people have trouble digesting lactose, even if they don't realize it. Cheese, ice cream, and other milk products can cause gas and runny stools. Pay attention to how your body responds to these foods and avoid them if they cause you distress, and in general keep these types of meals to a minimum.

**Caffeine.** It's a stimulant, which is great for perking up our brain, mood, and energy levels, but also the muscles in our digestive tract. That's why so many people poop within about an hour of drinking a cup of coffee in the morning—the caffeine speeds up peristalsis, the muscle movement in our intestines that scoots the poop along and eventually out of our bodies.

Now, some people love the reliability of the laxative effect a cup of coffee brings to their morning routine. It allows them to get their daily poop out of their system at a relatively predictable time every day and frees their butt and mind to enjoy without fear whatever delights the day may hold. But drink a strong cup or several not-so-strong cups throughout the day, as many people do to keep themselves alert, and your chances of needing to go to the bathroom or even shitting on your partner during sex will likely go up.

On the other hand, you could also find yourself with the opposite dilemma of constipation, because while caffeine is a stimulant, it's also a diuretic. Translation: it makes you pee. And if you're peeing a lot, the fluid that should be entering your colon to help your poo stay soft and move along is instead being eliminated into the toilet. You definitely don't want that. So make it a rule of thumb that for every cup of coffee you drink, you consume an extra glass of water during the day in addition to what you normally consume. You can also make some small changes to your caffeine consumption. For example, if you turn to coffee throughout the day to keep you going, try switching to espresso and dark roasts, which have less caffeine per serving. You could also make a brew of half caffeinated, half decaf. Or switch entirely to decaffeinated coffee. Despite the name, there's still caffeine in the product, just not as much as in its fully caffeinated form. Even heavy coffee drinkers who consume three or more cups of caffeinated coffee per day don't generally notice any withdrawal symptoms when they switch to decaf.[23]

**Artificial sweeteners.** Unlike sugar, artificial sweeteners and sugar alcohols aren't rapidly absorbed and used for energy, leaving them to ferment in the gut where they can cause gas and bloating. Some have such a strong laxative effect that the FDA requires them to be accompanied by a warning.[24] Beware of diet drinks and no-sugar versions of your favorite packaged foods and beverages.

**Fructose.** That's the sugar found in fruit, and too much fructose can give you the runs. Fruit should absolutely be a part of your diet, but don't go overboard, even in summertime when the cherries are to die for.

**Alcohol.** It's an irritant and it contains a lot of sugar and carbs, which, as we've learned, our digestive tract doesn't appreciate. In addition, it too, like coffee, is a diuretic. You know how alcohol makes some people's face flush red? That happens because they can't metabolize a certain byproduct of alcohol, which builds up in the system, dilating the blood vessels and turning their faces red. The same dilation and flushing process happens in your ass when you drink. Combine dilated veins with the uninhibited behavior and impaired judgment that can follow a night of drinking, and you make it much likelier for a bottoming session to result in pain and even damage, including the development of hemorrhoids.

Some of the best nights of our lives often start out with an excessive meal, endless refills of liquor, and a decadent dessert. I would never want anyone to give these things up. Besides, not everyone responds to these delights the same way. But optimizing better gut health and motility never hurts, and it gives you information that you can use to make the most informed decisions possible.

## CAN I BOTTOM IF I HAVE AN AUTOIMMUNE DISORDER OR DIGESTIVE CONDITION LIKE IBS, IBD, OR SIBO?

People with inflammatory bowel diseases, autoimmune issues, or other conditions that cause chronic diarrhea or otherwise give them stools full of water or mucus are frequently under the impression that anal sex isn't an option for them. But it is! With some care and precautions, and lots of communication with partners, many people with these conditions enjoy an active anal sex life. Ideally, patients like these should insist their autoimmune specialists, gastroenterologists, and nutritionists coordinate their care to ensure all aspects are well managed and work together to help you control your symptoms. This will necessitate you being forthright about your sexual history and activity. If you need advice on how to discuss these issues with your doctor, or even how to find a doctor who will be sensitive, compassionate, and respectful, go back to review chapter 3.

You're likely already mindful about what you eat, but by further analyzing your diet (for example, you may be asked to keep a food journal), lifestyle, and levels of stress, your doctors will hopefully be able to help you find patterns to your flare-ups. You'll want to discuss the optimal amount of fiber you should be ingesting, as too much or too little can wreak havoc on your system. Talk to them, too, about adding probiotics to your diet. Once you know your triggers, you'll be able to avoid them when you're planning on enjoying some anal, and minimize the risk of feeling gastrointestinal discomfort at an inopportune time.

Some IBS patients who take semiglutides like Wegovy or Ozempic for weight loss or sugar control find that it also allows them better control over their bowel movements. People with IBS often can't evacuate their bowels fully when they poop, which means they constantly feel like they have to take a shit, compelling them to make repeated mad dashes to the bathroom. With the better muscle control and more compacted stools as a result of the semiglutides, they're able to fully empty their bowels, which leaves them feeling more comfortable, and more confident for anal sex. The anatomical rules of where poop is stored and how and when it descends apply to you, too. You don't have to be more afraid than anyone else of pooping during sex unless you're having an IBS flare-up with symptoms.

———

You can't go wrong by following the recommendations in this chapter. Ultimately, the diet and nutrition for an optimal gut won't just improve poo quality and motility, but will also positively affect all other aspects of your health. Eat for health and nutrition, but always eat for pleasure, too. What makes you feel healthy and vibrant will also make you feel sexy, which is definitely good for your anal sex life!

When your diet and nutrition is well balanced and fine-tuned to your needs, you'll find that the most effective cleaning regimen will be, quite simply, going to the bathroom. No matter how much you improve your diet, or how committed you are to taking your pre- and probiotics and supplements, the risk of a little streak of poo here and there will never get to zero. So there's one more thing you can do to minimize the risk. It's something you were probably going to do even if I advised you not to, which is why I insist that you learn to do it correctly, because most of the time, it's this most popular pre-anal sex cleaning routine that's usually responsible for the shit shows that often follow. Folks, it's time to talk about douching.

## CHAPTER 7

# Douching—Less Is More

I've been a part of the community long enough, both as a gay man and as a physician specializing in anal medicine, to know that no matter how much evidence there is that diet and good nutrition are the healthiest cleansing habits to ensure a bowel-free butt, most bottoms are going to clean out their asses, and most tops are going to expect it of their bottoming partners. With the exception of those who enjoy a certain kind of kink, no one, including me, wants their anal fun accompanied by even the smallest side order of poo. So we douche. For the uninitiated, that's the act of spraying a solution up the butt to rinse it out before sex. I'd prefer to use the term "anal cleanse," but almost everyone calls it douching, so that's what we'll call it here, too.

**TOP TIP:** Trust me, your bottoming partners are doing their best. But sometimes in their eagerness to get perfectly clean they overdo things, and so you see a little excess liquid, or maybe a substance that looks like mucus. It's a shitty thing, but it happens, and it's unhelpful to make a big stink about it. Our job as tops is to be supportive and understanding. And if you really want to keep it from happening again, read this chapter (and the last one, too!). You can be a part of the solution, helping educate your partners and the bottoming community so that everyone can just relax and enjoy themselves.

The unfortunate thing is, everyone's doing it, but nobody actually wants to. My patients complain about it all the time. Douching is a huge chore. It's time-consuming. It's anything but a turn-on to see shit coming out of your ass, even when it's happening in private. Then after spending an hour in the shower they head out, hemorrhoids flaring, water dripping out of their ass (at least, they hope it's just water), feeling bloated and gassy, and in the end, they sometimes *still* shit on their partner! That is, assuming their anxiety doesn't get so bad they bail on intercourse altogether. It's just hard to feel sexy when your mind keeps turning to the possibility of poo. Yet despite the douching ritual's imperfections, we all return to it time and time again because it's still the only way most people can get even close to feeling clean before an anal encounter. We do it, but not with joy. Worse, when we're not doing it for ourselves but because we know it's expected, we do it begrudgingly. It just sucks, because prepping for sex is supposed to be fun, adding to the anticipation and excitement, like foreplay to the foreplay.

And I think it can be. See, the reason douching is so annoying and unpleasant is because most people do it incorrectly, in many cases unwittingly setting the stage for utterly craptastic results. Case in point, one of my patients, let's call him Eric, and his partner decided to invite a third party, a young "Adonis," into their bedroom. When Adonis arrived, Eric, a self-proclaimed "seasoned bottom," gave him a clean douche bulb and showed him the way to the bathroom so he could freshen up. When the guy was done, Eric took his place in the bathroom to do his own cleansing routine, leaving the new man and Eric's partner to get things going with a little foreplay. And they did. By the time Eric opened the bathroom door, his partner was planted face-first into the Adonis's ass, rimming him with all the enthusiasm of a dog with a Puppucino. As Eric stared agape, a loud fart trumpeted over the men's groans of pleasure, and next thing he knew, brown liquid was spewing violently out of his third's ass. You'll recall that Eric's partner's face was…right there. Milliseconds later, the liquid was replaced by something with the texture and color of mud, hitting Eric's partner square in the face and his open mouth.[1]

Your worst nightmare, right? But this shit didn't have to happen! None of the horror stories I've heard—of people pulling out of their partner and a full BM following, or of people coughing or sneezing and filling their Calvins with "poo water"[2]—were unavoidable side effects of anal sex. No. They were self-inflicted side effects of ineffective, incorrectly executed anal sex prep. That isn't anyone's fault. Even the most popular social media videos on this topic aren't recommending best practices, leading us to use the wrong solutions and the wrong delivery methods at the wrong time with the wrong amount of volume and force. Combined, these mistakes can create the perfect conditions for the shitty scenarios we're trying so hard to prevent. In addition, there are more reasons to learn to douche correctly that go far beyond sparing you or your partner from embarrassment or a case of shit-dick. The same habits that make douching such a drag can also negatively impact your anal health and future bottoming joy.

## BACK TO THE BOOTY BIOME

Researchers suspect that douching can lead to higher incidences of HIV,[3] STIs,[4] and anal injuries such as bleeding[5] or inflamed, irritated hemorrhoids in people on the receiving end of anal sex. Why?

You'll remember that the rectum is just a conduit for poop, connecting the holding tank of the sigmoid colon to the anal canal chute through which poop is expelled out of the body. The only time stools might linger in there is when you feel the urge to poop but hold it instead of going to the bathroom. Otherwise, shit don't sit—once you poop, the rectum is empty. All clear. The only feces left in the rectum shortly after a bowel movement might be a few traces along the organ's walls here and there. Those rectal walls are lined with a layer of mucosal cells, and those cells are coated with mucus and the healthy bacteria that comprises the microbiome in the butt.

Now, when we douche, we do potentially wash away any lingering traces of poo that might be left behind along the rectal walls. But at the same time, we're also washing away that mucosa and disrupting the booty biome. With that microbiome altered, the lower numbers of good bacteria present can allow harmful bacteria to proliferate. If you've ever suffered from diarrhea or experienced a yeast infection after taking an antibiotic, that's why—the drug altered the microbiome of the gut or vagina to the point of causing an over-proliferation of bacteria or fungus.

The same thing can happen in the rectum and anus. Depending on the type of douching bulb you use and how you insert it, what kind of douching solutions you use, and how frequently you use them, you can cause real damage to your rectal lining. Scrape away that top layer of rectal lining, and beneath is a raw layer of immature cells that aren't as able to resist trauma, leaving you with little left to defend your fragile bum from viruses and infection. Add in the effects of toys, cheap lubes, wet wipes that wash away protective skin flora, condoms, or literally anything you introduce into the anus, including just a hard penis, and you potentially launch a bacterial disequilibrium that can set off a cascading set of problems in the ass, even for someone who follows a fiber-filled diet and takes pre- and probiotics specially made to protect the booty biome. This is likely why the few studies conducted on this topic indicate that people who douche show higher rates of infections, illness, and injuries.

Our microbiome is as unique as a fingerprint, with its own baseline for homeostasis and equilibrium. Yet while each of us carries our own universe of bacteria, with every interaction we share and exchange them. Sharing our microbiomes doesn't always translate to illness or negative repercussions, but some people are more sensitive to certain bacteria than others. There's just no way to know how our bodies are going to respond to each other, even if we believe we're in good health.

## THE BETTER WAY

It's not just one particular aspect of douching that can be troublesome. You could use a just-right solution, but use the wrong kind of bulb and cause a problem. You could use the perfect bulb with a different solution and cause a whole other problem. Safe, effective douching requires a specific set of tools and technique. We can't control our body chemistry, and we don't always know when we're carrying potential irritants to our partners, or that we're susceptible to unknown irritants ourselves. We can only control what we put into and on our bodies. As we move through the following steps to douching, I'll critique common practices, break down why certain options aren't ideal, and examine what improvements are available so you can make the most educated, optimal choices.

I realize this is a controversial move. I've been accused of perpetuating poop-shaming and bottoming stigma because I spend so much time teaching people the best ways to douche. I've been told that by acknowledging the general desire for shit-free sex, I'm putting additional pressure on bottoms to get spanking clean. Respectfully, I call bullshit. I know my people. I know that feeling clean is a key component to feeling sexy. I've learned that no matter what I say or what they know rationally to be true, people will still insist on douching. Spend five seconds in a chat room or any forum where people can ask questions or express their fears anonymously, and you'll see that the pressure to perform is already there, the anxiety and stress over poop is real, and people are willing to try all kinds of inadvisable, harmful tactics to guarantee cleanliness and avoid embarrassment. I can't stop people from douching, but I can meet them with compassion and encourage safe, effective practices. If I can even get you to just douche less—for sure skip it during your dilating sessions!—I'll consider that a win for all of us.

In the anal community cleanliness is next to godliness, and if that makes you quiver, I'm all for it. Bathe in your Tom Ford shower gel. Banish that Taco Bell breath. And by all means, keep your bottom clean. But there is a better way. For twelve years I've listened to my patients, analyzed the pitfalls they fall into, and thought about what I could do to minimize everyone's time spent douching while reducing risks, maximizing pleasure, ensuring you leave the bathroom feeling sexy and confident with a slick, clean, fresh-as-a-daisy hole. What follows represents the end result, a protocol that delivers the clean outcomes you want in little time.

As we discussed in the last chapter, if you've had a bowel movement recently and don't feel any urge to poop, you're probably clean. The fact is, because poop doesn't linger in the rectum, douching is unnecessary and not a requirement for good, spontaneous anal sex. So if this isn't a topic that concerns you or is keeping you from having or enjoying anal sex, it's the one chapter I give bottoms permission to skip. You won't hurt yourself or hurt anyone else if you don't douche. In fact, it would be better if you didn't.

Did you hear that? My company makes and sells douches, and I'm telling you, you don't need them. How 'bout them apples?

If you are going to douche, however, or want to learn how, there is a right way and a wrong way. The instructions in this chapter will have you douching effectively, efficiently, and safely.

## THE TIME IS RIGHT WHEN IT FEELS RIGHT

How far ahead of time you need to douche before having anal intercourse, or whether you choose to have anal intercourse at all on any given day, is a subjective, personal call that requires a deep understanding of your body's natural rhythms and your own comfort levels. In a perfect world, I could draft a recipe where instead of telling you to preheat your oven, I'd say, "Forty-five minutes to two hours before having sex, retreat to the bathroom with a douche bulb and solution." Yet that doesn't help the person whose evening starts with happy hour at 5 p.m. and ends in the sheets at midnight, or the one whose phone lights up at 2 a.m. with, "U up?" Every scenario and everyone's needs are going to be different. What works for you might not work for me, and vice versa.

When Eric's Adonis showed up for their anticipated ménage à trois, Eric ushered him immediately into the bathroom with a brand-new douche bulb, and thirty minutes later a shitstorm ensued. Was that an example of cause and effect? Maybe. Common sense says that if someone starts stimulating your ass minutes after you squirt water up there, it might trigger a bowel movement, especially if you're using incorrect tools and techniques. And yet, maybe not. If you've been eating a fiber-rich diet, taking supplements, and dilating regularly, your butt is probably good to go for sex even without douching, or if you decide to douche only fifteen minutes beforehand. If you haven't adopted those eating and nutrition habits and stuck to them regularly, you should probably plan ahead a little more and build in time for anal prep before letting another person near your hole. If you ate three slices of pepperoni pizza for dinner just a few hours before accepting a pre-dawn booty call, you might want to stick to some outercourse—rimming, mutual masturbation, frottage, etc.—instead of engaging in penetration. There's no right answer. That's why we've talked so much about anal anatomy, correct pooping practices, diet and nutrition, and why I want you to work on improving that business before getting down to this business. So before you start douching, check in with yourself and take stock. How do you feel? Is your body up for this? If the answer is yes, let's get it on.

## WHAT YOU'LL NEED

For all the reasons I listed earlier, douching is often thought of as a necessary inconvenience we have to get through in order to get to the good stuff. But when you follow my instructions, just as dilating can become part of your regular self-care, douching can be a sensual precursor to foreplay. It's a built-in moment alone to slow down, enjoy your body, and anticipate the pleasures in store. So much of good sex happens in the mind—use this time to let your imagination roam.

Speaking of dilation, before you even attempt douching, you should have completed the six-week dilating protocol outlined in chapter 5. No, seriously. Please don't insert anything into your hole until it's been properly trained and conditioned, and you have a general idea of your comfort level and capacity. Once you can comfortably take the medium-to-large size dilator, you can integrate douching should you wish to.

For the love of all that is hole-y, do not ever, EVER insert something that has been in your ass into your mouth or, for our AFAB friends, into your vagina. No matter how clean you are down there, there is always bacteria present, and you run a high risk of getting sick or contracting an infection if you cross-contaminate. AFAB people, it's the same reason why it's important to always wipe front to back after going to the bathroom.

With that said, we're ready to start.

Douching requires very few tools, but the type and quality of those tools matter a great deal. Here's what you'll need:

## A douche bulb

Many people assume that when it comes to purchasing a tool meant to get you clean, bigger is better, and the market is filled with large bulbs that promise to spray you with the force of Old Faithful. Don't buy them. When it comes to douching, less is more. Why? First, as we discussed earlier, large amounts of water, especially when applied repeatedly, strips the anal wall of its protective lining and upsets the rectal microbiome, making us more vulnerable to microcuts, tears, infections, and disease. A common practice is for people to repeatedly insert and reinsert the bulb, filling themselves up over and over again until they expel a clean stream of liquid from their ass. This constant assault of friction and fluid can make the delicate anal lining raw and irritated, which for obvious reasons isn't a great starting point for awesome anal sex, no matter how much lube you use later.

Second, jetting such large amounts of liquid repeatedly distends the rectum. This is especially likely if you use something called a shower shot, an ill-advised enema system you can attach to your shower, which doesn't always provide a way to regulate the water pressure. Now, the rectum has an impressive capacity to stretch. I've heard of someone taking in a vintage glass two-liter Coke bottle. (You're probably wondering, was it full or empty? I want to know, too.) Drug mules and smugglers use their rectums like internal duffel bags to carry cell phones and bricks of cocaine. Doctors have extracted bowling pins and peanut butter jars from their patients.[6] The rectum is tough. Yet if you overstretch its capacity, you stress the organ, and it can tear, or worse, cause significant laxity and incontinence. At minimum, unlike an overly swollen stomach that shrinks once you start eating less, the rectum doesn't snap back once it has been distended.

Some people's vigorous douching habits eventually cause them to *have* to rely on propelling strong jets of water into their ass in order to defecate. They douched with such intensity and frequency, they not only distended their rectum and weakened the inner muscles' ability to contract, but they also burned out the nerves and damaged the pooping reflex. The condition can compel people to bear down so hard to try to poop, they suffer rectal prolapse, in which the lower end of the rectum gets pushed out the anus.

Overdouching exacerbates other medical issues, too. Many people aren't even aware they have a common condition called diverticulosis, in which little pouches (diverticula) form along the weak spots of the colon walls. Spraying liquid onto and around those pouches can cause them to become irritated, inflamed, and even infected, a painful condition called diverticulitis with symptoms such as fever, rectal bleeding, and diarrhea.

The final problem with overdouching is that when you use that much force, even if you're just shooting several milliliters up your ass with one strong squeeze, you're inevitably pushing the fluid past the rectum, beyond the kink and into the sigmoid colon. You'll recall that's where the poop sits until enough builds up to trigger the body's reflex to defecate. Push liquid far up enough to get into the sigmoid colon, and you create the conditions for a poo mudslide, setting yourself up for a far bigger mess than if you'd never tried to clean yourself at all (this may have been the lesson Adonis learned). For this reason, I strongly advise against shower shots, because they can be inserted so much farther up the ass than a regular douche bulb. That's what's happening when you douche once, and you feel clean, and then you do it one more time for good measure and you expel a waterfall of poo. I've heard of people spending hours in the shower waiting for the water they expel from their ass to finally run clear, not realizing that their constant high-pressure, high-volume douching is making it impossible. The irony is when they finally do leave the bathroom after all that intense "cleaning," they've actually primed themselves to have a bowel movement. On top of that, their hemorrhoids are probably activated. The chance that the sex they were prepping for is going to be awesome is now pretty damn low.

If you're a porn star, into fisting, or really ambitious insofar as the large objects you choose to insert deep into your butt, it's possible that you need a deeper cleanse than the average person. But if you're just engaging in run-of-the-mill anal sex, your goal should be to simply rinse off the walls of the rectum, not subject yourself to a colonic. Think rectal bird bath, not car wash.

So, with all that said, what type of douche bulb *should* you choose? You want a small bulb with a tip not much longer than two inches, which is all it should take to get past the internal sphincter muscle, and a reservoir capable of holding two to three ounces of liquid. It may not stroke your ego as much to purchase an itty-bitty bulb instead of something that could rinse out a rhino, but your bottom and your sex partners will thank you.

## An isotonic, iso-osmolar douching solution

Isotonic? Iso-osmolar? What the hell does that mean? And why do I need to know? You need to know what it means so that you understand why the products you're otherwise most likely to use will increase your risk of introducing pain, complications, and trauma to your ass. You should know by now that I'm never going to tell you to do something or not to do something without offering you a solid reason, and this time is no different. So let's get our science on.

Quick super-simplified chemistry review: Osmosis is the process of water flowing through a permeable membrane. Tonicity refers to how much solute—particles—are in a solution, which affects the concentration of water in that solution. Place two different solutions together separated by a membrane—like an anal cleaning solution and the watery contents of a cell—and osmosis will occur. A solution that's *hyper*tonic (has more stuff in it than its neighboring fluid, so a lower concentration of water) and *hyper*osmolar will draw water out of a cell through the cell membrane; a solution that's *hypo*tonic (has less stuff in it than a neighboring fluid, so a higher concentration of water) and *hypo*-osmolar will cause water to be drawn into a cell through the cell membrane.

So an *iso*tonic, *iso*-osmolar solution is one that matches your cells' natural chemistry so that there's no reaction at all to its presence. When bathed in this neutral solution, the cells neither lose water (dehydrating them) nor gain water (causing them to swell), thus allowing the solution to wash freely over the cells without inflicting any harm. Why does that matter? Because the vast majority of people who douche use one or two common solutions that can damage the cells of the anal canal and ruin its delicate lining. Those common solutions are enemas and water.

**Enemas.** Many people assume that because enemas are designed to make poop flow freely out of the asshole, they can be used to clean out that asshole before sex. But enemas are designed to liberate poop from constipated asses, not well-functioning ones. Commercial enemas—whether phosphate, saline, glycerin, or coffee—are all formulated to soften any rock-solid masses stuck in your butt by pulling water into the stool. Where does this hyperosmolar solution pull that water from? The rectal cells. When that happens, a cell becomes dehydrated, and it dies. Now think about how many cells come into contact with that solution.

Damaged cells might not be an issue for a person who doesn't expose their ass to items from the outside world, but it does pose a risk for bottoms. For someone using the enema as intended, that is, for the occasional bout of constipation, cell death shouldn't be a big deal because the body has time to rehydrate and grow new cells in between uses. But if that person engages anally, and has sex after giving themselves an enema with someone carrying an STI, they're exposing a raw, open anal surface to that pathogen, making it that much more likely to get infected themselves. And if people with active anal sex lives are using enemas two, three, or more times per week to prep for sex, that doesn't give the body time to regenerate those cells, so the protective mucosal lining is constantly sloughed off and the cells underneath left exposed. (Hint: Your body will try to compensate by quickly producing more mucosal protection, so if you ever feel like you're cumming out of your ass, you're either overdouching or you have an STI.)

The danger is especially real now that condom use is dramatically lower than it used to be.[7] Only around one-third of men who have sex with men (MSM) use condoms regularly,[8] down from 78 percent of the gay and bisexual men engaging in anal intercourse in 1987. It's also half the number of all men who engaged in anal sex at that time.[9] Those rates have surely been affected by the availability of PrEP, but the use of PrEP is anything but universal, with enormous racial, economic, and geographic disparities among who takes it. In addition, PrEP is only as effective as the consistency of the person who uses it. Even if you take PrEP exactly as intended and prescribed, you may not be vulnerable to HIV, but you are still exposing yourself to other illnesses. That's a lot of people around the country at risk of disease before we even factor in the added risk of anal cleansing. Multiple studies of men who have sex with men who also clean themselves out with enemas report a higher incidence of HIV and other STIs. It's also worth noting that more research needs to be done to determine if it's actually the enemas creating the opportunities for these diseases and infections to take hold, or if people who cleanse with enemas also exhibit riskier sexual behaviors that expose them to more pathogens and harmful bacteria than people who don't use enemas.[10] For example, a booty biome disrupted out of equilibrium because of the overuse of enemas can allow for the overpopulation of the bacteria called Prevotella, which can alter the butt's homeostasis enough that it weakens the body's ability to fight bacterial infections and diseases. However, the rectal microbiome of men who receive condomless anal sex from other men can also reveal Prevotella overgrowth.[11] Anything that goes up the butt can cause some disruption of the anal microbiome and trauma to the rectal cells, but since you have a choice, don't choose enemas.

**Water.** In a 2018 study of MSM who douched, up to 93 percent of them did so with a liquid other than a commercial product specially formulated for rectal use, the most common being water.[12] And why not? It's pure, it's natural, how much damage could it cause? That's what people are thinking when they empty a store-bought enema and replace the solution inside with water. Clean off the tip of the bulb after each use, and you can refill the enema dispenser for free any time you want. No harm done, right?

Wrong. Unfortunately, water isn't benign when it comes to anal cleansing. We've talked about what happens when an enema solution—which is hyperosmolar—draws water out of the cell. A water solution does the opposite. It's hypo-osmolar, meaning instead of drawing water out of cells, the solution causes water to rush into the cells and flood them. Once the cells swell and their equilibrium is overwhelmed, they burst like water balloons. The cells die. This isn't a big deal if you're only occasionally shooting water up the ass, but if you're getting some play on a regular basis and douching with water every time, you're not giving those cells enough time to regenerate. Now your ass has lost its protective lining and experienced a permanent change to its microbiome, which can allow for harmful bacteria overgrowth and make that area extra vulnerable to STIs, viruses, and injuries like tearing. Add in water-based lube—made hyperosmolar because of the added glycerin necessary to make it work well—and you're really compounding the problem.

In the end, whether you're using water and flooding the anal cells until they explode, or using enema solutions and dehydrating them until they shrivel, these common cleansing routines are damaging to your anal health, and in the long run they can compromise your ability to successfully and enjoyably bottom.

## WAIT, SO WHAT *SHOULD* I USE?

Again, "nothing" is a perfectly good option here. However, if you do want to douche, the ideal rectal cleaning solution would be one whose composition was exactly like your anal cells' own, therefore able to clean the area without either dehydrating the cells or swelling them until they burst. In scientific terms, an isotonic, iso-osmolar solution. Until recently, that formula didn't exist. Since no one else was stepping up to develop it, I decided to try. I remembered that early in my career when I worked in a trauma unit, we used replacement solutions to help grievously injured or sick patients, in particular to resolve something called third-spacing, in which fluid leaks from a patient's blood vessels into other spaces where it doesn't belong, causing swelling (edema). When administered intravenously, the replacement solutions, which are dense and heavy, use osmotic pressure to draw that leaked fluid back into the blood vessels where it can improve a patient's blood pressure and heart function. Despite improvements made in the years since I worked in hospitals, these solutions don't always succeed, and sometimes they even cause third-spacing themselves. However, my understanding of their evolution and how these solutions were *supposed* to work helped guide my thinking as I developed a cleansing product that mimics rectal cell chemistry so well, it doesn't cause any disruption on contact. Unfortunately, the one we sell at Future Method, available in ready-made form or in powder packs you mix with water, is still the only formulation that fits this description.

My goal isn't to sell you more product. As I will say loudly from the rafters as many times as possible, douching is *not* a requirement for fulfilling anal sex. Having a better understanding of your anatomy, increasing your fiber intake, and adding pre- and probiotics should get you the clean results you seek. But if you're going to douche anyway, I want you to do it in a way that minimizes risk. If you don't have an isotonic, iso-osmolar solution available and need to choose between an enema or water, skip the enema. Use tap water instead. No need to boil it. However, don't compromise on the type of bulb you use. Keep it small.

Meanwhile, I'm just gonna take another opportunity to point out that many people get irritated from douching no matter what solution they use, which means before they even have sex, they're starting out with a raw, inflamed ass. Take my advice and at least try skipping the douche a few times once you've got your diet in optimal anal-sex shape. You probably already have so much other shit to worry about; I'd love for you to free yourself from worrying whether this particular kind is going to fuck up your fucking.

---

### Dr. Goldstein's To-Douche List

Okay, you've got your small bulb and your isotonic, iso-osmolar solution (either in ready-made form or powder pack; both work great), or a few ounces of water, at your side. You're ready to begin.

---

If after everything you've read here you really would like to skip douching, but you still need some peace of mind, there's something you can do to gauge how likely it is you've got any reason to worry about poop. Generously lubricate your asshole and a small dilator or any small toy of your choice, and gently insert it into the anal canal. Now remove it.

Do you see poop streaks? If not, you probably don't need to douche and can skip to step ten, then start your dilation steps to warm up for sex. If you do see some poo, or if you believe better safe than sorry, move on to step one.

There's another great benefit to pre-dilating before you douche—pre-dilating means pre-lubing! While less is more when it comes to douching, more is more when it comes to lube.

1. **Clean the tip of your bulb with warm water and soap.** (Do this even if it is the first time using the bulb.)

2. **Assemble the bulb and tip, then draw the solution into the bulb.** Be cautious and try to do this in one smooth movement to minimize how much air gets into the bulb. No one wants more gas in their ass!

3. **Apply an ample amount of lubricant to the bulb nozzle.** Yes, even if you pre-dilated with a dilator or toy.

4. **Assume the "Captain Morgan" position.** Stand with one foot resting on either your toilet or the edge of your bathtub. This position uses gravity to naturally help prevent any liquid from going into your sigmoid colon. Remember that the anal canal and rectum is where run-of-the-mill sex is happening. By standing upright, it helps you focus exclusively on that region.

5. **Slowly insert the bulb nozzle into your rectum. Keep it perfectly straight.** Be careful not to insert the tip at an angle or rub up against the rectal wall, which can create irritation, tears, swelling, or bleeding. I've had patients who used long, insufficiently lubricated nozzles who caused their own hemorrhoids that then developed into a painful condition called a fissure, which is basically a tunnel in the flesh of your ass.

6. **GENTLY squeeze the bulb**, allowing all of the liquid to flow into your rectum in a slow, steady, continuous stream.

7. **Continue to squeeze the now-empty bulb—do not release!—and remove both the bulb and tip from your anus.** This is to prevent backwash from entering the bulb.

8. **As soon as you've removed the bulb, expel the solution from your rectum into the toilet.**

9. **Check the water you've expelled from your rectum.** It's probably clear, and if it's clear, you're clean. If not, flush and try again. One or two more rinse cycles will probably do the trick. If it's getting laborious, it may not be your day to bottom, and you might want to re-evaluate your process. Is your bulb too big? Are you jetting too much water into your rectum, or doing it too forcefully?

10. **Disinfect the bulb by removing the tip and washing both tip and bulb with warm water and soap.** If you are jumping here from using your dilator to test how clean you are, wash it the same way. Rinse well.

More than once, I've had patients come to me over and over with the same STI infections. They tell me they're faithfully following the treatment I prescribe, the STI disappears, but then it comes back just a week or so later. How are they getting reinfected so frequently? I'll ask them if they're thoroughly cleaning their douche bulb or anal toys, and they'll say sure, they run it under water and rub it with a little soap. Then, at my suggestion, they'll go home and separate the bulb from the tip or any removable parts from the toys. They'll find them full of gunk, the perfect breeding ground for bacteria. Once they start cleaning their bulb properly each and every time they use it, the STI infections stop.

11. **Dry bulb and tip thoroughly with a lint-free cloth, or allow to air dry.** Store them in a clean, dry place until your next use.

And that's it! When you're done douching, start your anal dilation protocol if you didn't lube and warm yourself up earlier. This part should be fun. If you're using a good cleansing solution, you'll be feeling a little slippery, slick, and sexy. Using your dilators or toys not only gets your ass primed and pre-lubed for sex, but it should also prove to you that you're clean when you see them coming out of you shit-free. It also helps get rid of any excess liquid and air that might have accumulated from douching, relaxes the underlying muscles, and lubricates the entire anal canal.

CAUTION: If you feel pain or see blood at any time while douching or doing your anal dilation, stop immediately and plan on enjoying some other sexual activity other than anal sex this time. You need to take some time off and heal before allowing anything up there again. Then reread this chapter and try again, making sure to dilate with lube beforehand, increase the amount of lube you use, limit how much air you introduce into the region, and pay close attention to the angle at which you're inserting the bulb and the force you're using to squeeze the water into the rectum. If the pain or bleeding persists, see a medical professional.

## LESS IS MORE

In the interest of preserving your rectal health, I'm going to ask you to try an experiment. The next time you're in the mood to play by yourself, or are practicing your anal dilation, don't douche first. Just use the (cleaned) toys or tools and see what happens.

Nine times out of ten, it's going to come out of your ass clean even though you didn't douche ahead of time. I want you to remember this the next time you're confronted with a chance for some spontaneous sex with no time to douche first. Douching isn't a requirement for poo-free sex. Its real benefit is in the way it eases anxiety and boosts confidence. The more you experiment on your own time to see how rarely you see poo, the more confident you should become.

Even so, I know that most people will insist on rinsing themselves out more than the recommended one time. So I want you to try another experiment, especially if you already douche regularly and have a healthy fiber intake and exercise regimen. Keep all those good eating and exercise habits in place. But the next time you douche as part of anal sex prep, make one small change: however many times you feel like you have to rinse to get perfectly clean, rinse one time less. So if you normally douche five times, do it for only four. When you expel the water from your ass, take note. Is it clear? Yes? Start your anal dilation or play with a toy. (As we've discussed, you want to do this so that you're pre-lubricated and your muscles loosened to decrease the risk of injury during intercourse.) What do you see? Probably nothing. At that point, you should feel confident enough to enjoy what comes next without stressing that your partner is going to see a little shit on their dick or dildo.

Keep notes on how this process goes for you. If you got the results you wanted this time, the next time you try, see what happens if you douche only three times. Is the water you expel still clear? Do the dilators come out clean? Yes? Great, make that number of rinses your new normal for now. When you're ready, try ramping down the number again. At some point, you're going to see where the number of times you douche does and doesn't make a difference.

Your goal should be to douche as few times as possible. There has been very little research invested in the issues surrounding anal sex, and those of us committed to resolving common problems with limited resources are often only able to make a dent in them, not eliminate them. Until then, the one thing we do know with certainty is that the least amount of douching leads to the fewest number of complications. Remember, gut before butt. Fiber + healthy diet + pre- and probiotics = firm, regular, "clean sweep" poops = less douching = healthier butt = better and more frequent sex!

Follow these steps and my recommendations, and the time-consuming process you once approached as an obligation should become a brief yet titillating opening act you get to look forward to before the exciting main event. From now on, if you're in the shower for an hour, it's because you're having so much fun alone or with a partner, you don't want to leave.

## RISKY BUSINESS

No matter how many preventative measures you take, sex of any kind always has an inherent risk. The good thing about so many people being on PrEP is that it requires regular STI screenings every three months, which is great for the community (and incentive for health practitioners and patients to push hard for increased investment in sexual health education and access to preventative healthcare). Yet all the risk reduction practices in the world won't bring that risk down to zero. We accept that. The same is true for poo, and we need to accept that, too. Have enough anal sex and eventually, no matter how well you clean yourself, one day there will likely be a little mess. Our culture has made us believe that it's the worst, most embarrassing thing that could happen. It isn't, which is why experienced, secure tops don't paint-shame their partners for something totally natural that comes with the territory. After all, plenty of tops have had a hard time getting it up or staying hard. Everyone has their off days. Compassion is an attractive trait.

**TOP TIP:** Some bottoms have suggested that tops who ghost them or cancel at the last minute should have to pay a cancellation fee to reimburse bottoms for the amount of time and money they spent douching to get ready for sex. If bottoms are douching the Future Method way, it's not a huge inconvenience or that big of a deal, but it's the principle. Tops, you might consider making a copy of this book or at least a copy of this chapter available to your bottoms in the spirit of helping them see that douching isn't necessary, but if they still feel compelled to do it, it shouldn't be something to stress over. It also indicates that you fully understand and appreciate their efforts to create the best sexual experience possible for both of you. And if that pre-sex bottom-cleaning ritual means that much to you, it would be a thoughtful gesture to keep douching solutions and instructions on hand.

The sooner as a community we stop shaming each other if a little shit makes it onto your sheets or your lover's dick or other playthings, the better for all of us. It's worth mentioning that Eric says that now that enough time has passed, he and his partner laugh about it. In the end, the hallmark of a good lover, and the greatest turn-on, is confidence, generosity, and an appreciation for everything the human body has to offer.

## CHAPTER 8

# The Real Deal

This is it! Your ass happily took the small dilator. It happily took the medium dilator. Maybe you're ambitious and went for it with the large dilator or even the cone, and that's been a good experience, too. You're ready for the next step. If you've followed all the prep protocols discussed so far—dilating, ideally with a glass dilator, and a cone; eating fiber-rich food and taking your supplements; and douching if you choose—there shouldn't be much left for you to do to get ready for your big moment except whatever makes you feel sexy, beautiful, and confident. You're now ready to learn all the ins and outs (hopefully followed by many, many more ins and outs) that comprise a successful, fulfilling anal experience for both bottoms and tops.

For bottoms, however, your lesson starts with this: Banish the idea that you're gonna get fucked. I mean technically, yes, you're going to experience penetration and pleasure. But no acrobatic sexcapade for you, my friend, at least not during the coital part of this session. In fact, you're going to go for the exact opposite. You might want to think about this first in-person experience less as sex and more as a continuation of your dilation training. What you'll do next is a bit like asking a friend to spot you at the gym, except while they're naked and hard (or wearing a strap-on).

## TAKE CHARGE

Many bottoms, especially men, have found themselves on the receiving end of pernicious stigmas and stereotypes labeling them as passive and weak. There's a cultural assumption that if someone is taking it in the ass, they're being taken. We're going to flip that script. When it comes to anal, and especially during these first attempts at anal penetration, the person with the dick, dick-like appendage, or toy isn't the star of the show. That honor belongs to the bottom.

As you finally do the deed, I want you to remember everything you learned over the past six weeks as you spent additional time alone and naked with your dilators, especially what felt good as you worked at your own rhythm in your own time. Because though you're about to invite another person to join you in anal play, you're going to set the rules of the game, and the rules should revolve around allowing you to recapture those good feelings you experienced on your own. It's imperative that you have a frank conversation with your partner. The best tops will be willing, even eager to read this book too so they can gain a thorough understanding of anal anatomy, pelvic angles, and the stages of relaxation necessary for pleasurable anal engagement. Regardless, ensuring that they agree to hand you the power and control over this sex act will be absolutely key to you enjoying a successful first bottoming experience. Even a born top in every sense of the term can find it freeing to give up control and surrender themselves to a new experience. Later, once you know what you're doing and have a better sense of what works and doesn't for you, you can share power. Heck, you may relish the idea of soon going full sub. You do you. But for now, your partner's job is to be a living, breathing dilator. Make sure they understand what they're getting into, literally and figuratively.

**TOP TIP:** If someone has invited you to help usher them into anal sex, take that responsibility seriously. It's not just a matter of respect and kindness, but of safety, especially if this is your first time, too. Be prepared to give up control and let them take the lead. Later, when everyone is comfortable and confident, and familiar with their limitations and desires, you can grasp the reins and ride as fast and hard as you both like. But for now, your job will be to keep your penis hard, your strap-on or toy straight, stay still, and remain supportive. The better this goes, the better allllll the sex with this bottom is going to go.

## CHOOSE WISELY

If you have a monogamous partner, presumably you've been using your dilators and toys to train your ass to receive whatever your partner has to deliver, whether it's a dick or a strap-on or they wanna get in on the dilator fun. Some people make the fun choice of ordering dildos in the shape of their partner's penis to use as dilators, thus making absolutely sure they can comfortably take the real deal when the time comes. If you don't have a monogamous partner and you need to choose someone with whom to share this moment, choose wisely. Sometimes people opt to launch their real-world bottoming selves at a sex party or group outing. This is a terrible idea, as it can allow other people to take control of the environment, the timing, and the pacing of the act. I've also sewn a lot of people up whose eyes proved to be bigger than their hole. I admire the ambition, but it's better for everyone when a bottom's first time is successful and satisfying from beginning to end.

If you're on the hunt for a dick, this is the time to be selective. Be careful when choosing partners from the apps; camera angles and filters can make it hard to know what size penis is really going to come through your door, and you need to remember your limits. After all that dilating practice, you should be acutely aware of what length and girth works best for you. Choose someone with a penis that's too big for your ass, and you take the obvious risk of tearing or straining yourself, or just being uncomfortable, every time you lower yourself onto them.

**TOP TIP:** If you're endowed with a particularly large dick—you know who you are—I promise you, too, will have infinitely better sex if you take your partner's needs, build, and anatomy into consideration than if you just ram yourself in with little thought to any of it. Take it upon yourself to prove you know what you're doing. Refresh your anatomy knowledge by rereading chapter 4 if you need to. Be generous! Generous with your encouragement. Generous with your foreplay. And super generous with the lube you put on their ass and your appendage. Be sensitive to your partner's facial cues and body language so you can respond immediately as necessary, and keep asking them the all-important questions: Does this feel good? Are you okay? What do you want me to do? Let them know you can be trusted, and encourage them to communicate what they're feeling. Make sure they know you're here for them, and that they don't owe you anything. If they need to take a break or stop and try another day, support them in that decision. Help make this a positive experience no matter what, so that you both look forward to the next time.

But choose someone who's too small, and every time you raise yourself up they'll be more likely to come all the way out of you. As you know from your training, once you get that dilator in all the way, even as you pull it back you never want it to completely leave the anus because every time you reinsert, you risk accidentally reentering at an angle that can cause pain or damage. So once it's in, it should stay in even as it moves back and forth. A penis that's too small can be poky and cause the same kind of pain if it hits you the wrong way.

This is the time to be picky. You need to be motherfucking Goldilocks and choose a dick that's not too big, not too small, but just right. And you need a partner you can trust, someone who'll follow instructions and do what you need them to, which is to say, not much. You're welcome to get them off afterward, but for the purpose of intercourse, they're the passengers on your ride.

## GET READY

As with dilation and douching (if you do that), make sure that you're in a positive frame of mind and feeling great as you get ready for this big moment. If anything doesn't feel right physically or emotionally—you're still feeling tight, you're nervous, you're stressing out about work, or you're having any doubts about your partner—call it off and try another day. The more care you take to ensure a successful first encounter, the more likely you'll be having countless more encounters in the near future. If you're feeling good, you're good to go.

## Gather your supplies

1. Your favorite condoms (if you use them)
2. A lube shooter
3. Ample amounts of your favorite lube (see page 91)
4. The dilators, cone, and/or toys you were using successfully throughout your dilation protocol
5. Special sheets you don't mind getting stained with lube, and even towels to protect the bed.

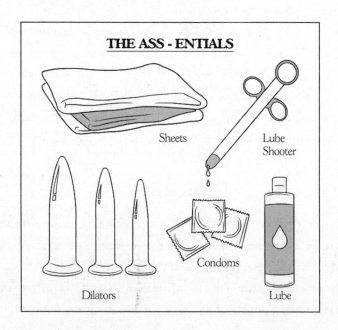

### THE ASS - ENTIALS

Sheets

Lube Shooter

Condoms

Lube

Dilators

## Predilate

Even if you're zealous about your routine and keep your anus stretched and fit regularly, you'll want to predilate with dilators, toys, a silicone cone, or even lifelike dildos before your first person-to-person anal session (this is true whether you're a noob or a pro). If you choose to let your partner be present, be strict—you should be the only person inserting anything into your hole. You can enjoy any good sensations that arise and arouse, but don't think of this particular session of pre-dilation as foreplay (though when you're not trying to insert anything into your rectum, of course you can indulge in other forms of foreplay, so long as it doesn't get you so wound up you can't control your body or movements. As you're about to see, self-control will be critical for being successful in this first round of anal sex). Later, you can absolutely incorporate dilation into your foreplay, but in this particular instance, think of it more as a warm-up exercise that requires concentration.

Whether you predilate alone or with a partner, the point is to stretch your skin and muscles and get some of that lube in place long before you need it, and to engage in conscious relaxation. Override the reflex to contract. Breathe deeply. Put yourself in a positive frame of mind. Take note of everything you experience. Is the dilator going in smoothly? Does it feel comfortable? Do you notice any bleeding? If all looks and feels good, you can move on to the real thing.

### LET'S DO IT!

You might be surprised to learn that I see very few injuries coming from the fisting community. Why? Because those people know that if they aren't extremely communicative with their partners, they could wind up in deep shit, literally and figuratively. You may not ever choose to try fisting, but when engaging in anal, I want you to talk as though you are. This is no time to be shy. It's not the time to be generous to your partner or worry about their orgasm. If you can't find a partner with whom you feel you can communicate directly and openly, without feeling self-conscious or fearing their judgment, you may want to turn to a dildo or a fuck machine for now. It's not even time to think about your own orgasm, though it's possible you'll have one. Your only goal for now is to get comfortable and build confidence by testing the relaxation and dilating techniques you've learned in a real-world setting. You're going to dictate every move of this dance with Beyoncé-like precision. And you're going to be vocal and forthright with your partner about what feels good and what doesn't so they know what you want. Don't leave anything to chance.

You may also be surprised to learn that you're not going to flip over on your hands and knees and present your ass to your partner doggy style. I know that's generally considered the anal gateway position, but in fact it's the worst entry to bottoming you could choose, whether you have a vagina or a penis. It not only prevents partners from being able to read each other's faces to gauge how much they're enjoying themselves (or not), it also gives tops complete command over the speed, depth, and angle of penetration. There's time for that later. In this beginner stage, it's the bottom who gets to dominate, and the bottom who determines how deep, how fast, and how soon they're ready to start experimenting.

Here we go!

1. Have your partner lie down flat on their back. Their dick, if they have one, needs to be fully hard by now. If your partner is planning to wear a strap-on, now's the time for them to strap in. Make sure your anus is slicked with lube, giving yourself one more hit with the lube shooter for good measure if you want. Apply a good amount of lube to your partner's dick or dildo.

2. Next, face your partner, who's still lying on their back, and straddle them in a kneeling position. Whether you call this pose the cowboy, cowgirl, cowpoke, or cowabunga— and for the sake of gender neutrality and fun, I'm going to stick with that last one—it's the position that will give you the most control over your position, speed, and depth of penetration. It's intimate, because you can look into your partner's eyes, but this also means it's ideal for good communication. Presumably you've picked a partner who cares that you're having a good experience. Straddling your partner face-to-face, you'll be able to better let them know when something feels good and when it doesn't.

3. Gently, slowly, lower yourself onto your partner, easing the dick or dildo into your anus. Just like you do with your dilator, you'll likely encounter some resistance as soon as you hit that first set of muscles, the external sphincter. Once you feel resistance, breathe, and hold your position for three to five seconds. That will give the muscle time to relax. Then pull all the way up and out, relubricate your

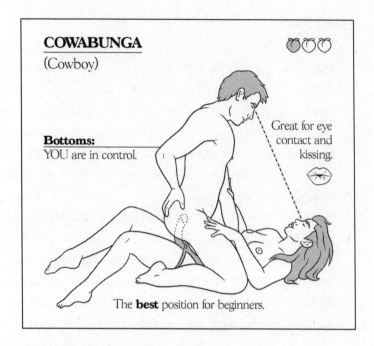

**COWABUNGA**
(Cowboy)

**Bottoms:**
YOU are in control.

Great for eye contact and kissing.

The **best** position for beginners.

partner, and do it again, exactly as you've been practicing during your six weeks of booty camp.

Inch your way down as far as feels comfortable, count to five (don't forget to breathe!), raise yourself up and relubricate once you feel any resistance or discomfort, especially when you hit the next group of muscles, the internal sphincter. Hold there for a few seconds, breathing and relaxing, before pulling out and starting over. Don't force anything. Remember, real dick or a strap-on attached to a human is going to be a change from a dilator or toy. You might feel the same sense of fullness you felt when you dilated, or it could feel different this time. You might find you have some limitations you didn't experience during training. That's okay. You're the one in control, and you set the pace. It can take as many as four to eight times to pass that third muscle and finally sit all the way down.

**TOP TIP:** These are the instructions from your perspective: Generously lubricate your dick or dildo, lie down on your back, and hold the phallus with your hand as still and steady as you can. Be patient as your partner works to relax, get comfortable with muscle one, two, and three, and settle down onto you. Think of yourself as a human cone. Remember, this is all about your partner for now. If this is your first time or you're nervous, it may be a challenge to keep a penis hard, but be patient and feel free to stroke yourself or do whatever it takes to keep things up. On the other hand, it could feel amazing, in which case enjoy yourself but stay calm and in control.

4. If you're able to comfortably take the entirety of your partner, sit there for a minute or so and take time to assess. If everything feels good and there is no pain, you can start to enjoy a very slow, careful ride. You should be doing all the work here, no thrusting from your top. As you move up and down, take note of the physical sensations you experience. As your excitement grows, your instinct may be to speed up. Try to resist that impulse. The slower you go, the better you'll be able to concentrate on your positioning and analyzing how everything feels. That said, if everything is super comfortable and you want to climax while being penetrated, go for it! Just be very careful. When you

orgasm, you reflexively squeeze your butt, which puts a great deal of extra stress and strain onto a poor ass that's already trying to cope with the stress and strain of being penetrated. The full-body convulsion of a climax means you could lose control, and could cause spasms, irritation, or additional trauma. Just keep trying to keep that phallus inside so there's less chance you get poked at a painful angle by your partner. If you do orgasm and feel discomfort, try dilating after sex to help you relax. If you're turned on enough to want to get off while being penetrated, but can't, dismount and finish off some other way. To get that aroused and not climax puts you at risk for complications like prostatitis. You gotta cum.

CAUTION: If at any point you feel pulling, stretching, tearing, stinging, or pain, no matter how minor, stop and dismount your partner. The same goes for emotional pain or discomfort. Seriously. Don't worry about disappointing your partner, or get embarrassed if you need to stop. This isn't a race or a competition. It's crucial that you enjoy a positive feedback loop so that once you do succeed, the next time goes even better. If this first anal encounter isn't successful, take a few days to rest and heal, then start back up with your dilating protocol for an additional week or so. For information on what might be the problem, as well as possible solutions and recommendations for how long to wait before proceeding, turn to chapter 9.

## AFTERCARE

Don't worry if your partner didn't climax inside you, or even at all. For this moment, you get to concentrate on your experience. Take note of how many tries it took before you were able to sit all the way down, what positions were easiest, and what sensations you want to revisit or never have again.

It's also totally okay if your first time didn't blow your mind. This first time with another person was really about getting the mechanics down. Besides, with a few exceptions, most first sexual experiences are awkward. It takes time and practice to get good at this, just like it took time and practice to get good at whatever other kind of sex you've been enjoying for most of your life. But hopefully you'll both be excited to plan another tryst soon.

Just as your bum needs to be treated gently before sex, it deserves some TLC afterward, especially one that's new to bottoming and that's sustaining some pressures it's just getting used to. You want to promote a healthy healing environment so that your asshole is always ready for the next go-round! Even after the best anal sex session, there will be some micro trauma, such as small tears. That's why even when things are going well, you don't want to indulge in anal sex every day in the beginning. Your body needs a few days to heal. In the meantime, a lot of people enjoy pampering their bum with cocoa butter suppositories, scrubs, and soothing creams. If things feel a little swollen or tender, try using some anti-inflammatory hemorrhoid cream like Preparation H. You'll want to follow these aftercare instructions after every sexual encounter.

If everything went perfectly and the whole experience with your partner is easy and comfortable, stop! Give yourself two to three days to relax and heal before trying again, *following the exact instructions you did this first time around.* Yes, I'm afraid I'm still not clearing you for sexcapades. I know it's a drag to continue in such a methodical, unerotic fashion when your body and mind are ready for the orgy scene in *Eyes Wide Shut* or pretty much any episode of *Euphoria,* but this is how you ensure that your ass is ready and your technique sound before moving on to a more advanced stage of anal engagement, and actual, full-blown sexy sex!

## TIME TO RAMP THINGS UP!

If you've completed two rounds of First Timer anal sex with no complications and no pain, my friend, you're cleared to start ramping up your fun, either alone or with partners. Go back to chapter 4 and refresh your memory about where to find those delicious erogenous zones we discussed, either the prostate or the A-Zone. Keep this book nearby so you can easily check it as you continue to gain experience, but eventually, with practice, you'll get to the point where you no longer need to take such a clinical, literally by-the-book approach. Enjoy acting out (carefully!) all the fantasies you've been dreaming of. Enjoy exploring the way different poses bring out your and your partner's(s') more submissive or aggressive tendencies, and let your play flow organically and fluidly. As always, the key to enjoying any sex is open and honest communication, and a little imagination! I've listed some ideas to help get you started.

## Have Fun with Foreplay

You'll recall that I discouraged you from thinking about pre-dilating as foreplay. That's because at that point you're doing it purely as a warm-up stretching exercise, not with the goal of arousal. I cautioned you about getting carried away with foreplay because I wanted you to stay focused while you were completing your first copulation. Once you've got the pre-dilating protocol and the mechanics of anal sex down and can engage without any complications, though, you can and absolutely should go back to whatever pre-sex play turns on you and your partner(s). Gentle touching, kissing, sucking, licking—do and ask for whatever sets your body on fire. All the signs of sexual arousal, like deeper breathing, sweating, and heat, indicate that your muscles are relaxing, and your blood flow is increasing. Indulge and revel in giving and receiving those delicious sensations. Take your time!

## Introduce More Toys

Use well-lubed dilators to your heart's desire, so long as only you control the insertion into your hole during your pre-dilation period. After that, feel free to enjoy them and other toys on your own or with partners, always remembering to lube, lube, and lube up some more. Some beginner favorites include:

### *Anal Beads*

Anal beads are a sex toy composed of a string of balls with a handle or grip on one end. In some versions, the balls are all the same size, and in others they start small and get bigger along the length of the toy. Many people enjoy inserting these into the rectum and then gently pulling them out. You want to be careful with these, though, as there is space between each bead, and if your sphincter gets swollen, it can make removal difficult (and in rare instances, impossible without medical assistance). If you're interested in trying them out, choose a strand where the beads are flush up against each other, which will provide pleasurable sensations as the beads move in and out of your body without the potential for irritation or discomfort. As always, start small and move slowly to avoid the risk of injury.

## Butt Plugs

Butt plugs are great for solo and partner play. Nowadays, you can get vibrating models, and even ones that can be remotely controlled by a partner, so you can enjoy anal play even while you're out and about. For beginners, I recommend finding one that has a tapered design (it'll resemble a cone) that allows for gradual insertion rather than a blunt tip. Note that despite what the name might suggest, they should not be left in for extended periods of time.

## Vibrators

Anal vibrators are like vaginal vibrators, except they are designed to stimulate the P-spot (in which case they're sometimes called a prostate stimulator or massager) or A-zone, and they have a base so they can't accidentally get sucked into the anus. They use vibrations to send waves of pleasure throughout the body, and can help intensify anal orgasms. Enjoying anal vibrators is less about repeated in-and-out movements and more about leaving the toy inside and letting the vibrator do all the work. At this point I probably sound like a broken record, but with these, too, start slow and low. Only increase the speed and vibrations as you feel comfortable. Just don't be surprised if your whole body shakes when you orgasm—it'll be *that* intense!

## *Dildos*

Anal dildos typically have a phallic shape like vaginal dildos, except they also have a base to help prevent them from getting lost inside the anus. They can range in size, girth, and material, and some even have lifelike features. Using a dildo is just like using the real thing. Just as when you use dilators, make sure you use copious amounts of toy-safe lube, start slow, and work your way up to your desired size to give your muscles and skin time to stretch and strengthen. If you're using dildos in between playtime with a partner, I recommend finding one that closely resembles your partner's member. That way, you're constantly training your sphincters to be able to accommodate this size, making bottoming more pleasurable for everyone.

It's worth a reminder when using toys (or engaging in any kind of anal play) if you or your partner(s) are AFAB, be extremely careful about moving between anal and vaginal areas. No one should touch an anus and then insert their hands or fingers into a vagina without thoroughly washing their hands in between. To do otherwise puts the vagina owner at risk of infection.

I also strongly advise that you only allow anal penetration with toys, strap-ons, and dick. It's just risky to let people insert their fingers. When they don't know what they're doing, or get too excited, they can accidentally poke an anus at weird angles that can lead to injury. Stick to butt plugs or toys that can't bend or scratch. Regardless, make sure anyone putting their hands or fingers near your anus has clean, clipped, filed nails! And if someone is stroking around there, ask them to put your lube to work, and reciprocate by using lube when touching your partner's penis if they have one.

## PLAY AROUND WITH POSITIONS

So what are the best anal sex positions? There's no consensus. What makes you see stars may send someone else to sleep. What rocks your world on a bed might leave you cold in a shower or the wall of a club dark room. Each position changes participants' pelvic angles, and one's height and weight can make certain positions more appealing with some people than with others. So can dick or dildo size and shape. Enjoy exploring the way different poses bring out yours and your partner(s)' more submissive or aggressive tendencies, and let your mood guide your play more organically and fluidly. As always, the key to enjoying any sexual position is open and honest communication. You can slowly start to share power, cede dominance if you wish, and give and take pleasure.

You'll remember from chapter 4 that one of the best things about anal penetration is that it indirectly stimulates the P-spot and the A-spot. Ideally, before allowing a partner to penetrate you, you'll have played around on your own to find these erogenous zones with a dilator or toy. Once you bring a partner into the mix, though, you'll have to adjust to the shape of their dick or strap-on shape. For example, ironically, a downward-facing dick or dildo isn't ideal in doggy style because in that position it can pound a bottom's prostate, which can be painful and even cause both prostatitis and blue balls (an inability to ejaculate). This is why it's paramount for all parties to be aware of their anal anatomy, and hold on to what they've learned about the alignment of the rectum and anal canal, the location of the sphincters, and the site of the P-spot or A-zone. However, in general, if a top owns or wears a cock that points upward, bottoms will experience the most pleasure (and least amount of discomfort) in face-to-face positions. If the top's dick faces downward, it's best to face away from each other to stimulate the P-spot and A-zone. If it ever feels like a top is hitting a wall, they probably are—either of the rectum or the pelvis—and repetitive penetration will cause discomfort and even pain. Make sure to communicate to avoid injury.

One item you might add to your essential accessory kit for partner play is a sex pillow or wedge. Available in a variety of shapes and sizes, these cushions are designed to support and facilitate most sexual positions, and bonus, help everyone enjoy themselves for longer periods of time without suffering any cricks, strains, or joint pressure. Unlike regular bed or throw pillows, they're generally made from a high-density foam that holds its shape and provides more direct support. They also come with a removable, machine-washable cover. Wedge-shaped styles are better for raising a bottom's hips, knees, or thighs, which help raise or lower the pelvic angle in such a way as to allow for easy, comfortable penetration. Ramp-shaped options are longer and larger in size, intended more for back support. Ramps and wedges are often paired together for extra fun play, and some come with "mounts," pockets where you can insert dildos or vibrators for hands-free penetration and stimulation. These pillows aren't just great for bottoms; tops enjoy them for the additional knee support and the way they raise bottoms (or other parts of the body) higher for easy penetrative or oral access.

What you'll find here are suggestions for both classic and kinky anal sex positions that anyone can get behind. We've ranked each on a scale of one to three peaches to help you know which ones are beginner level, which are good for people with a little more experience, and which are advanced. Only one position gets a single peach rank, though—the cowabunga. It's the only position beginners should use, and it's the one that ideally you will start with every time. All the other positions are ranked intermediate or advanced. Each has its pros and cons, and whether you enjoy them will likely depend on you and your partner(s)' level of experience, height, and flexibility. As always, go very, very slowly as you experiment and never stop communicating. With so many options, you'll be sure to find one and hopefully more that work well for everyone involved.

**TOP TIP:** Now that your bottom has got the hang of things, you can start to engage more actively and play! The rules still apply, of course. Use tons of lube, talk to each other, and always keep your knowledge of the anatomy of the ass and rectum front of mind so that you don't inadvertently hurt your partner. Have fun!

## Reverse Cowabunga

This one is similar to the traditional straddling position, except the bottom faces away from the top. More advanced and flexible

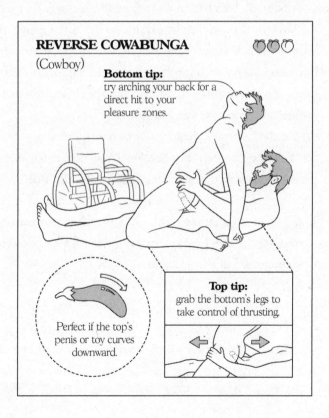

**REVERSE COWABUNGA**
(Cowboy)

**Bottom tip:**
try arching your back for a direct hit to your pleasure zones.

Perfect if the top's penis or toy curves downward.

**Top tip:**
grab the bottom's legs to take control of thrusting.

bottoms can spice things up by laying back on top of their partner's chest, after which the top can grab the bottom's legs and use them to take control of thrusting. This also allows the bottom to be a little more submissive while still enjoying literally being on top.

### PROS/CONS/TIPS

- Because most penises are either straight or curve upward, it can be difficult to achieve prostate stimulation in this position because the penis will most likely be angled toward the bottom's tailbone, which is opposite from the prostate. As a result, the bottom can potentially experience posterior pelvic pain because the penis may be repetitively hitting a wall of tissue.
- Bottoms can try arching their back and adjust how they're sitting on the penis or dildo to make sure it's as direct a hit to their pleasure zones as possible.
- While the bottom is technically in control in this position, the fact the partners are back-to-front can make it more challenging to read visual cues and to communicate.

**When you're done trying this or any other position that strikes your fancy, don't forget to take time for the aftercare outline on page 183 of this chapter.**

## Missionary

Based on the virality of their social media posts, straight women, or at least the ones watching the Amazon Prime movie *Red, White, and Royal Blue* in 2023, were surprised and delighted to learn from a scene in the gay rom-com that two men could enjoy missionary-style sex. Well, why not? This is a great position for *anyone* craving intimacy, and can be as "vanilla" or spicy as your mood dictates. The bottom lies on their back with their legs spread apart, either in the air, wrapped around their partner, or with their legs up against their chest, while the top penetrates from above. To give tops easy, direct entry into their anal canal, bottoms can adjust their pelvic angle by arching or flattening their back (like a cat-cow yoga pose you'd normally do on your knees). Then, once the top is comfortably inside, the bottom can adjust the height of their legs up or down to play with fit and sensations.

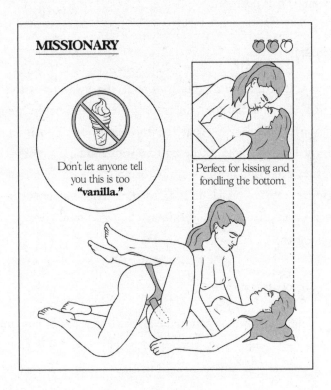

**MISSIONARY**

Don't let anyone tell you this is too **"vanilla."**

Perfect for kissing and fondling the bottom.

## *PROS/CONS/TIPS*

- As a more top-dominant position, it's a nice next step once a bottom feels comfortable handling variations in speed and depth of penetration.
- Because you're face-to-face, you can create great communication and elevated intimacy. The position also allows the bottom to manually pleasure themselves (or let their top do it for them).
- If your top is pegging, pulling your knees up so your partner can scoot closer will make it much easier to successfully enjoy this position.

## Doggy Style

This one is iconic, with the bottom facing away from the top on all fours, and the top penetrating them from behind, either standing or kneeling so that the top's penis or dildo is in line with the bottom's hole. If the bottom wants to take a more active role, they can grind up against the top and help with penetration. Beginner bottoms need to avoid doggy style, but once they've gained experience and can relinquish being in total control, it's a hot classic.

## *PROS/CONS/TIPS*

- Height differences can make all the difference in how much partners enjoy this one, especially if you're pegging, so

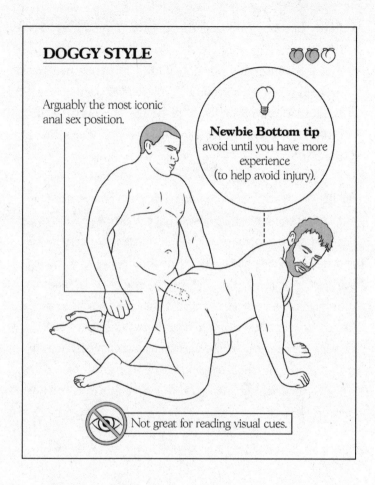

## DOGGY STYLE

Arguably the most iconic anal sex position.

**Newbie Bottom tip**
avoid until you have more experience
(to help avoid injury).

Not great for reading visual cues.

explore using pillows and furniture to get everyone aligned comfortably, whether the top is thrusting upward, downward, or straight in.

- Penetration in this position can feel harder and deeper, which some bottoms love, and others don't.

- Many bottoms find that this position is good for prostate stimulation.
- Tops! Because this position allows for deep penetration, proceed with care so you don't injure your partner.
- Because the bottom tends to be more submissive in this position, it also requires a lot more work and stamina from the top.

**TOP TIP:** Once you and your partner are in the groove and comfortable with anal, it can be easy to get carried away in this position with rapid, vigorous, or "rough" thrusting. Be very careful and stay in control, because if your partner bounces too enthusiastically and moves the goal, or you lose your aim and ram your dick into something more solid than their hole, you could literally break your dick. A common result of penile trauma is Peyronie's disease, in which scar tissue develops and forces the penis to curve, no longer allowing it to develop a full erection. It's a painful condition and requires early intervention to keep it from getting worse.

## The Spoon

Another sensual and intimate option, especially for bottoms. Both partners lie on their sides, with the top on the outside acting as the "big spoon" while penetrating the bottom—the "little spoon"—from behind. For an extra deep penetration, the bottom can adjust their legs so that the top can achieve more direct penetration. It's the best of both worlds, allowing for cuddling and cumming at the same time.

# THE (double) SPOON

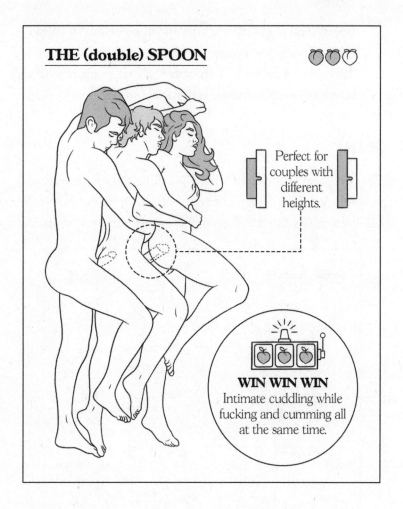

Perfect for couples with different heights.

**WIN WIN WIN**
Intimate cuddling while fucking and cumming all at the same time.

## *PROS/CONS/TIPS*

- This can be an uncomfortable position for either party depending on the length and natural curvature of the top's penis or the design of the dildo.
- It's really good for people of different heights.

- Sheets tend to get stained after spooning because both partners are lying down during intercourse (worth it!).
- This one is a favorite for the way it allows partners to enjoy simultaneous penetration and manual stimulation.

## The Arch

This is another variation of what I'm calling the cowabunga, and should be reserved for experienced bottoms with flexible backs. The bottom sits face-to-face on the top, but instead of placing

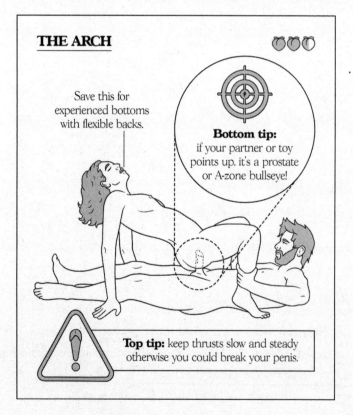

**THE ARCH**

Save this for experienced bottoms with flexible backs.

**Bottom tip:** if your partner or toy points up. it's a prostate or A-zone bullseye!

**Top tip:** keep thrusts slow and steady otherwise you could break your penis.

their knees on the bed, they plant their feet on it. Then the bottom leans back. At this angle, the penetration can be intense, especially if the natural curvature of the top's penis or the dildo faces up, which will be a direct hit for the prostate, if the bottom has one.

## *PROS/CONS/TIPS*

- This position is extra stimulating for both tops and bottoms.
- The bottom needs to move slowly and gradually, and keep their thrusts slow. Otherwise, they could break their partner's penis if they possess one.
- Tops with penises sometimes find this one uncomfortable because it limits the range of the bottom's pelvic angle.
- Both parties may find it hard to achieve pleasure if the top has a penis that's rigid or curves upward.

## The Bodyguard

Sometimes you don't want to take it or give it lying down. The bodyguard is essentially doggy style with both parties standing up. This is a great position when both partners want to be active because it doesn't limit either party to resting on a piece of furniture. You can do it wherever you want so long as you have great balance or can hold onto something sturdy nearby (like a wall, table, or sink). As with doggy style, the top is usually in full control, so this position should be reserved for experienced players only.

# THE BODYGUARD

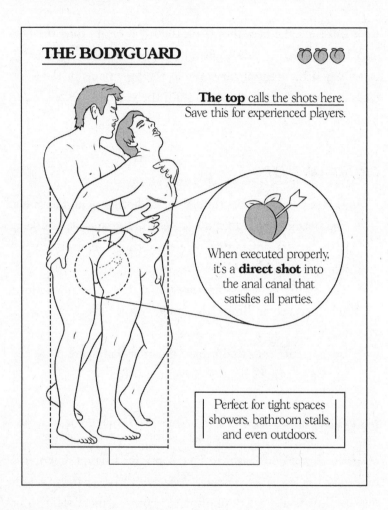

**The top** calls the shots here. Save this for experienced players.

When executed properly, it's a **direct shot** into the anal canal that satisfies all parties.

Perfect for tight spaces showers, bathroom stalls, and even outdoors.

## PROS/CONS/TIPS

- This position can be tough on tops and bottoms if there's a big difference in height between them. Doing it successfully may require someone to crouch or stand on tiptoes to ensure direct access between the penis or dildo and the asshole.

- When done right, it allows for a direct shot into the anal canal and can be very pleasurable for both parties.
- This is a great position for tight spots, like a bathroom, shower, or outdoor areas where lying down isn't a good option.

## Pirate's Bounty

Similar to missionary, but way sexier. In this position, the bottom lies down on their back with one leg down and the other raised in the air or resting on the top's shoulder while they're being

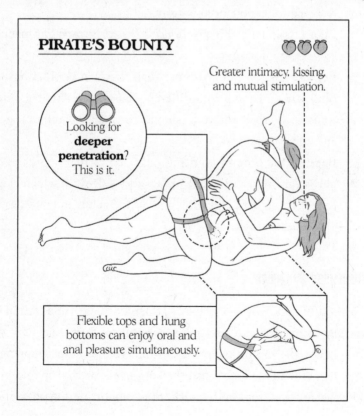

**PIRATE'S BOUNTY**

Greater intimacy, kissing, and mutual stimulation.

Looking for **deeper penetration**? This is it.

Flexible tops and hung bottoms can enjoy oral and anal pleasure simultaneously.

penetrated. This position is ideal for bottoms who want to give their tops deeper reach, for the farther up and back the top can push the bottom's leg, the deeper the top can thrust. A flexible top paired with a long-schlonged bottom can sometimes orally pleasure their partner while inside of them!

## PROS/CONS/TIPS

- Similar to missionary, this position gives the top more control over the speed and depth of penetration, so it should be reserved for experienced bottoms.
- Like missionary, this position allows for greater intimacy, kissing, and fondling.
- Because the top can go deeper than they can in other positions, they may tap into different sensations—some good, some bad—so the bottom should constantly communicate and adjust as necessary.
- Because the bottom is lifting only one of their legs, their pelvis can tilt, causing the top to hit a side wall, which can hurt. Lifting both legs will even out the pelvis and may provide a better angle.

## Suspended Congress

Meant for the serious and seriously athletic, strength and stamina are key to making this position successful for everyone. Facing each other, the top picks up the bottom. Rather than wrapping their legs around the top's waist, the bottom allows the top to support their thighs from underneath, thus supporting the bottom's hips against the top's pelvis. Either partner should feel free to lean up against something sturdy, like a wall or window, for balance and support. But if the top is feeling strong and ready for a challenge, they can try moving away from the wall.

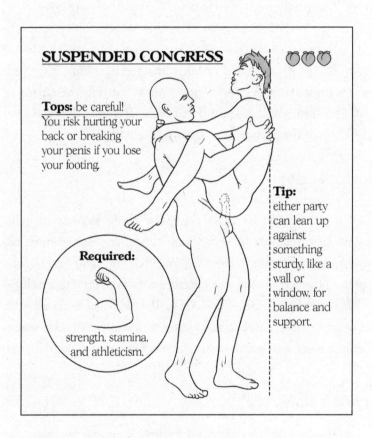

**SUSPENDED CONGRESS**

**Tops:** be careful! You risk hurting your back or breaking your penis if you lose your footing.

**Required:** strength, stamina, and athleticism.

**Tip:** either party can lean up against something sturdy, like a wall or window, for balance and support.

## PROS/CONS/TIPS

· For tops who can pull this off successfully, they can skip the gym that day and not feel guilty!

- The top needs to have a good awareness of the bottom's pelvic angles—keeping everyone at the right height and angle of insertion are critical to make this position fun for everyone.
- This position gives tops more control than any other position, and they need to take that responsibility seriously. There's a lot riding on their shoulders (and penis or dildo).
- That said, compared to other anal sex positions, it's in this one that the top is at most risk of hurting their back or breaking their penis, if they have one, should they lose control of the bottom or their own footing.

## Bumper Cars

Not recommended for new bottoms, this one is pretty complicated. If you're both fit and flexible, however, done right it will make sparks fly. The bottom lies on their stomach, legs slightly spread. The top, facing the opposite way, positions themself on all fours with their penis or dildo in line with the bottom's hole. It not only looks hot, but also creates new and exciting sensations because it engages couples at angles most don't usually experience.

### *PROS/CONS/TIPS*

- This one can be dangerous for both tops and bottoms. Not only can a top break their penis, but because of the angle, an AMAB bottom can damage their prostate if thrusting gets too aggressive.

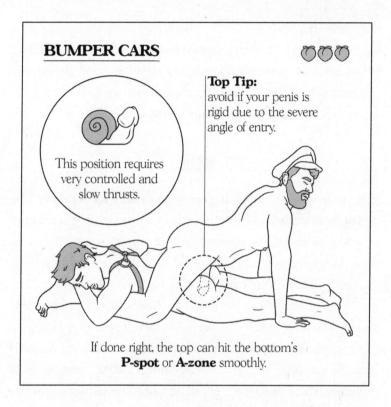

**BUMPER CARS**

This position requires very controlled and slow thrusts.

**Top Tip:**
avoid if your penis is rigid due to the severe angle of entry.

If done right, the top can hit the bottom's **P-spot** or **A-zone** smoothly.

- Tops need to proceed with a very controlled and slow thrust, and their movement will be somewhat limited.
- If done right, the top can hit a bottom's prostate smoothly. Not to mention, this position is exceptionally great for breeding.

The same rule is true for these positions and any others—if you experience any discomfort, stop. And if you do have to stop, all is not lost. You're naked, your partner is naked, you've made the time—if you're still in the mood, just switch to some other kind of play with the promise to try anal again another day. Just remember that front-to-back rule: never put something that was in a butt in a vagina, mouth, or near the eyes without thoroughly washing it or changing the condom first.

## DEBRIEF

Especially when you're just getting to learn what you like and don't like, what works easily and what's still a challenge, take the time to talk about your experience with your partner once you're done. What did you love? What did they? What would you both want to do again? What do you think you could do to succeed the next time in a position that didn't work as well as you'd hoped it would? Would toys help? How about a better pillow?

And while you're at it, don't forget to check in with yourself. How do you feel? You've just stepped into a whole new world of experiences and sensations. It can be a heady experience. Do you think you might want to revisit some of those questions posed in chapter 3 about your identity and what you like and don't like? That's cool! In fact, that's what this is all about—exploring, evolving, and embracing every facet of who you are.

## KEEP IT UP!

The best bottoms bottom regularly, if not with partners, then solo, two to three times per week. You know that feeling when you skip the gym for a couple of weeks and then you drag your-self back? It sucks, and it's usually disappointing to see how much ground you lost, and hard to face how much you're going to have to work to get it back. It's the same with bottoming. Especially in this beginner phase, you want to be sure to keep exploring all the pleasures of your hole with new positions, new lubes, and new toys. You've done everything to work your ass into bottoming shape—don't lose all your progress. Make another date with your partner soon if you have one, and dilate often in between.

# PART III

# AFTERCARE

## CHAPTER 9

# When Things Go Wrong: Injuries and How to Fix Them

Hopefully by now you're a pro, sailing through dilation protocol, regularly getting enough fiber, and having steamy, satisfying sex when you want to. Still, no matter how careful you are, if you choose to bottom, at some point in your life something isn't going to feel quite right. Or your partner will tell you something looks different back there. Or you'll go to the bathroom and... ouch! It's a bummer, but it's normal.

I've had to coax a lot of people off the ceiling because they think an injury or an STI diagnosis means the end of their anal sex life, or even their entire sex life. But that's just not true. These complications are just the nature of this particular two-backed beast. And you know what? Even people who *don't* have anal sex or engage in butt play can develop some of these conditions or suffer injuries and infections. All of the common problems we'll cover in this chapter—tears, symptomatic hemorrhoids, skin tags, anal gland abscesses, fistulas, scarring, and rectal prolapse and looseness—can affect anyone who has an ass.

If you were unable to successfully dilate or bottom, or if you did one or the other and are now experiencing any kind of pain in the butt, you should find enough information in this chapter to help narrow the possibilities of what could be going on, learn about some over-the-counter initial treatments, and guide you when discussing your symptoms with your health care provider.

If you've been dilating or bottoming and everything feels fine down there so far, or if you're reading this book to educate yourself before embarking on the anal road, even better! The more you know, you know? Familiarizing yourself with the potential pitfalls and problems associated with anal will help you more quickly identify what's possible to treat at home, and when you need to seek professional medical advice.

**TOP TIP:** Tops, anyone with an ass can find themselves on the receiving end of anal pain, swelling, irritation, itching, or other discomfort, so it will behoove you to read along. In addition, if you're a top because you've often found it too uncomfortable to bottom (a possibility you were given a chance to think about back in chapter 3) you may find the solution in this chapter. What if what's causing you pain is a hemorrhoid, and a simple procedure could get rid of it? How would that open up the possibilities of your sex life? Imagine if the little skin tag or bumpy scar that makes you feel self-conscious were gone. Would that change things for you?

Even if in the end you're content being a top, it can only do you and your partners good if you're as aware of the injuries that can befall a bottom as they are. And if you see something, if you've read this chapter, you'll have good, helpful information to pass on so they can heal it quickly, and you can get back to fucking.

---

## When to Seek Professional Medical Care

I know how things work in the real world. Most people don't run straight to the doctor the minute they feel a little pain, itchiness, or rawness. They assume the problem is temporary, they look online for easy at-home remedies, and they ride the symptoms out until they heal on their own. But if symptoms haven't improved after three to five days, get yourself to the doctor. I can't tell you how many people come to me informing me they need help treating a symptomatic hemorrhoid, when in fact they've got a rip-roaring infection.

It's important to read through this entire chapter to learn what symptoms you might experience, the most common anal ailments, and what treatment options are available, as some are specific to our anal communities, meaning general proctologists may have little to no knowledge about them. In addition, if you wind up needing surgery, you'll want to make sure it's done correctly the first time. Sexual wellness practitioners with expert understanding of anal sexual issues do exist and are available, but depending on where you live, you may need to seek them out via telehealth and/or travel. But know this: your hole and your bottoming game are worth the effort and deserve the best management. Help is out there. You can find a list of resources in Appendix C at the end of this book.

While I hope the information in this chapter should help guide you whether and when you need a doctor, I do want to be clear that it is *not* a substitute for consultation, diagnosis, or treatment with a licensed medical professional. The information I provide in this chapter (or anywhere else in this book) should not be used to disregard medical or health-related advice from your physician or care team.

## SYMPTOMS: ACUTE OR CHRONIC?

Anal injury symptoms can run the gamut from pain, burning, itching, and bleeding. You might be able to feel swelling, extra skin, or a tear. If you spot small traces of blood or feel a little pain immediately after dilating or having sex, see spotting on the toilet paper when you have a bowel movement after doing either, or notice a small amount of discharge, don't panic. It doesn't necessarily mean anything serious is going on. In fact, the intensity of symptoms doesn't always track with the severity of the problem. Harmless issues that quickly go away on their own could hurt a lot at first, whereas an injury that needs medical treatment could cause you almost no discomfort at all. More important is to pay attention to when the symptoms occurred, how quickly they resolve, and whether they reoccur.

While correlation doesn't necessarily equal causation, the first thing to think about is what might have triggered the symptoms (doctors sometimes call this the inciting incident). It could be anything. You dilated, you had sex, you used less lube than normal, you took bigger dick than usual, you tried a new position, you were constipated, or you took a humongous shit, and ever since then your bum has been in a little pain and felt out of sorts. Maybe you try some over-the-counter treatments (I recommend some good ones below), and after a few days, your butt feels better. Now, pay attention to what happens next:

1. Nothing hurts the next time you go to the bathroom or resume anal sexual activity. Problem solved!
2. You feel no pain when you have a bowel movement, but the very next time you dilate or bottom, the symptoms return.
3. Shitting and fucking still hurts all or most of the time.

By paying attention to the timing and duration of symptoms, you're figuring out whether the symptoms are acute or chronic. Acute symptoms come on abruptly, but then heal and don't reoccur. Chronic symptoms persist or recur over time. Acute symptoms that aren't treated properly or don't heal all the way can become chronic. Knowing whether your symptoms are acute or chronic isn't about determining their severity, but help you point to the cause and track how well the healing process is going. If your symptoms come and go, you may be treating the symptoms appropriately, but not addressing their underlying cause. If you can poop fine, but you still can't resume your normal dilating and sex habits, you may have healed enough to handle the pressures of shitting but not enough to get your ass back to comfortably taking the extra pressures of anal sex. Should you decide it's time to see your health practitioner, being able to tell them if your symptoms are acute or chronic will help them diagnose your problem more quickly, especially if they have a limited understanding of or experience with treating issues that can arise from anal sex.

Insofar as when to see your health practitioner, if you think it is at all possible that you've been exposed to a sexually transmitted disease (STI), make an appointment as soon as possible. You don't want to sit on that shit. Early treatment is always preferable.

## EASE YOUR SYMPTOMS IMMEDIATELY

In the short term, what do you do if you experience any symptoms like mild pain, discomfort, burning, itching, bleeding, swelling, or soreness? Start by taking a break from dilating or sex to give your body a chance to heal. In addition, over-the-counter (OTC) treatments are available that can help speed that healing process and give you symptom relief, allowing your anus to rest even as it copes with the normal pressures of physical activity and bowel movements. In many cases, chronic problems often start out as acute ones that would have remained one-offs if they'd been treated appropriately with OTC remedies. The treatments suggested below are easy to follow and can often head off more serious, harder-to-treat problems at the pass.

Now you might be thinking, hold up, Dr. Goldstein, before we move on to treatments, what *is* this? What are my symptoms telling me? Hell if I know; only your doctor can tell you that for sure. Regardless, trying any or all of the OTC remedies below is a recommended first step no matter what the cause is. And if your symptoms compel you to make an appointment with a doctor who diagnoses something that requires prescription medicine or surgical treatment, they, too, will likely suggest you use OTC remedies for initial symptom relief. So there's no harm in starting them as soon as you feel discomfort, even before you know for sure what's causing them. In fact, many anal sex practitioners regularly use these treatments as prevention tactics before and after all of their sex training and play, from dilation to toys to the real deal. A little preventative TLC never hurts.

## Epsom Salt Baths

Epsom salt baths can provide relief for inflammation, soreness, swelling, and muscle pain. Readers of a certain age may have spotted milk-carton size boxes of this stuff in their grandparents' bathroom cabinets. Cheap and recommended to ease all kinds of ailments from muscle soreness to arthritis, Epsom salts aren't actually salt at all; they just look like and dissolve like it. They're chemical compounds made up of magnesium and sulfur (Epsom is the English town where the compound was first discovered in the water). While scientific studies are inconclusive, people have long reported getting relief from aches, minor pain, and stress after soaking in warm Epsom salt baths. They provide two major benefits: (1) they chill you out, and (2) they can help increase circulation, which means more local blood flow to the anal region, which is soothing and encourages healing. Follow the instructions on the package of salts, using comfortably warm water in the bathtub. I recommend taking at least two a day (more if you'd like). Make sure your ass is fully submerged in the water. If possible, hold your cheeks open to maximize the skin's contact with the Epsom salts. Splash your hole!

## Stool Softeners and Laxatives

If you feel any irritation or see a little blood after sex or bowel movements, there could potentially be a microtear somewhere in the lining of the anal canal. It could be a cut or tear in the anus. The challenge is that no one can swear off pooping for the amount of time it would take for the skin to heal entirely; the wound splits again every time the skin stretches to accommodate a bowel movement. The answer—for this issue or any soreness, swelling, or pain—is to keep your stool very soft and your bowel movements easy so your skin doesn't have to stretch much. If you're already following an anal-friendly diet and good hydration practices, your stool shouldn't be too hard as it is. But if you want to make it extra soft (not runny), you can drink even more water, at minimum sixteen extra ounces, and adopt a bland, soft diet for a few days while continuing to take pre- and probiotics. You can also add over-the-counter stool softeners, like Colace, which increase the amount of water drawn into your stool, making it easier to pass.

Some people fear the pain so much they avoid going to the bathroom, which can then make them constipated, which will make shitting hurt even more. All the suggestions for softening stools apply, but you can also add over-the-counter laxatives. A gentle one is Milk of Magnesia. Another option would be Miralax. If you're constipated, add a capful of Miralax to a glass of water or juice, while continuing to take stool softeners three times per day. Keep this up for one week to ten days until you no longer see blood when you wipe, and then you can titrate back down. Stop the laxative first, then take one less stool softener per day, and add fiber and probiotics to your diet. Fun fact, if you're constipated, a big burger, shake and fries—none of which have much fiber, but do have a lot of fat and grease—can also get things going again. I understand many of us in the anal community want to control our fats and carbs, but indulging every now and then is a good thing, and this is a good excuse.

## Preparation H Cream

If you're experiencing any rectal itching, burning, swelling, or irritation, and especially if in addition to these symptoms you see bright spots of blood in your stool, on the toilet paper, or in the toilet bowl after a bowel movement, you can try a topical anti-inflammatory hemorrhoid medication. The most common brand is Preparation H, found at any pharmacy without a prescription. Many variations exist, such as ointments, creams, suppositories, and cooling gels, and all of them will do the trick, but I like to recommend the cream. If you're in pain, choose the one that also contains the numbing agent lidocaine. Careful, though! I've noted that many people can develop allergic reactions to lidocaine, especially if used for a prolonged period of time, so do a quick skin test on the inside of your wrist before slathering it to the inside of your ass, lest you be up all night with an itchy, red rash.

If you don't have a reaction, at night before bed and after each bowel movement, lube up the tip of the applicator and slowly, delicately insert a few centimeters of product inside the rectum (the applicators aren't very long). It should go in easily. Once you reach the end of the applicator (where it's attached to the tube), stop, and then gently squeeze a small amount until you feel a wet or cool sensation in the area, making sure to coat the outer rim of your hole as well. Remove the tip, then properly clean it according to the instructions on the box.

If it feels like your symptoms are higher up or deeper inside, the suppositories will probably be a better choice than the cream.

## Calmol-4 Suppositories

I'm like Oprah with these. You get a suppository! YOU get a suppository! Everyone gets a suppository! I think Calmol-4 suppositories are life changing, especially when used in conjunction with other remedies like Preparation H and Epsom salts. They contain cocoa butter and do a fantastic job at soothing the inside and exterior of the rectum, coating the anal lining to allow comfortable bowel movements when you're experiencing any of the anal symptoms we've mentioned. They're an over-the-counter product, but this brand is more commonly found at mom-and-pop pharmacies and online than in most big-name pharmacies. If you can't find them locally, order them online, and use Preparation H suppositories until the Calmol-4 ones arrive. I recommend using these at night, before bed and post-poop. Leave them in a cool area (even the fridge) as they can easily melt, especially in warmer months or climates. Pro tip: Before inserting the suppositories, pre-lubricate the area with Preparation H cream. This should make insertion extra easy, especially if you're experiencing some discomfort. Some people like to shower or bathe and leave their ass wet to let the water in the hole region make it extra easy to insert the suppository.

If during the first few days it's too painful and there's no way you're sticking anything up in your hole, even something tiny, don't fret. Just do all the other steps, and each day you can try again to see if you can handle inserting the suppositories. Always insert gently, but you will need to use a little bit of pressure to pop them past the last internal anal muscle and into the rectum. Read the instructions on the box carefully, especially if it's your first time using them.

## Gauze

Roll a strip of 4×4 surgical gauze into a cigarette shape and place it between your butt cheeks up against your hole. Not only will this absorb any bleeding or mucus and keep the lotions and creams you apply in place, it's also a great way to save your expensive underwear and sheets from getting stained. I tell my patients to use lotions and suppositories, along with the gauze, for three to seven days, then when everything starts looking and feeling better, start tapering off. The creams and lotions help with pain management, but once you're through that stage, the wound needs to dry out. Change the gauze every two to three hours to keep any mucus from sticking to the wound and keeping it moist, which would prevent healing.

## TEST YOUR RECOVERY—SLOWLY

Use your OTC treatment for one week and see how you feel. Bowel movements should be pain- and blood-free. If symptoms resolve and you feel better, let another week go by with no treatments and make sure there's no recurrence. All good? Great! This would be the benchmark for success if your goal was to only use your ass to eliminate waste. But if you're a bottom, the real test is whether the injury reoccurs the next time you try to receive.

After your two-week treatment and rest period, start over with your dilation protocol (see page 99), beginning with the smallest size. Test the waters and see how everything feels. If you can dilate with the small size and feel no pain or discomfort over the course of a session or two, advance to the next size. Again, see how everything feels over a few sessions. Keep things slow and steady, and keep evaluating. You're testing to make sure the site of the wound, which has now healed or scarred enough to withstand a normal bowel movement, is strong enough to hold up under the pressure of sexual activity. If you can go through your whole dilation protocol several times painlessly and problem-free, you can slowly and carefully try having sex again, reintroducing the size of dick or dildo that has never caused you distress.

If your anal encounter goes well and feels like a success, congrats! Looks like your acute symptoms have healed. Go on your merry, sexy way. Play to your heart's content.

But if you feel pain again, if you see blood again, if the discharge persists, if you just can't get comfortable—bummer, it means you've developed a chronic issue. It still might not be anything serious, but you need to get evaluated. Something is keeping your ass from being able to handle penetrative sex, and you need to get to the bottom of it. It's time to see a medical professional.

You'll need to be honest with your doctor. For example, if you came to me complaining of pain or discomfort that started during your dilation training, that would lead me down one diagnostic path of possibilities. If you dilated successfully and only started feeling symptoms when you tried sitting on a real, live partner, that would suggest the problem is something else. If your symptoms cropped up only after years of repeatedly and successfully taking dick or dildo, that would send me down an altogether different path. And if you're still feeling these symptoms after trying the OTC remedies above, that tells me something, too. The context of how and when you got hurt, how long the symptoms have lasted, and how they've responded to initial treatment will matter as much to your diagnosis as the nature of the injury or illness itself.

## COMMON PROBLEMS AND SOLUTIONS

We're going to look at the six most common challenges that can affect people who engage in anal sex—anal fissures, hemorrhoids, skin tags, abscesses, fistulas, scarring, rectal prolapse, and looseness. Again, the information presented below is not intended to help you self-diagnose, but to educate you about the possibilities so that you can better self-advocate and make the most of your time with a health care provider. All are treatable, but whether these injuries can be resolved medically or surgically will depend on multiple factors.

## Anal Fissures

Fissures are the most common injury I see. A fissure is simply a fancy word for a tear. As we discussed in part 1, the skin of the anus is thin, especially in women, which is why dilation training is necessary in order to be able to bottom. You have to relax and stretch the muscle and skin before subjecting it to the pressure of sex, or the skin will split. You've heard me talk about microtears. They're little cuts in the ass, sometimes visible, but sometimes so small you can't see them. They're the equivalent to the microtears you cause when you floss your teeth. In the same way that your gums will feel sore and bleed after flossing if you haven't done it in a while, then not hurt at all once flossing becomes your daily routine, microtears make your butt hurt and bleed because it takes time for the skin of the anus to toughen up enough to handle the pressures of sex. Fissures are bigger, badder versions of microtears. Symptoms include bleeding, pain (in general and during sex), discharge, burning, irritation, and sometimes uncomfortable sphincter spasms during and after defecation.

It's not just the force of sex that can tear the skin, but also poor lubrication, an awkward position, or the diameter and length of an item inserted into the anal canal. Penetrative sex isn't the only thing that causes fissures, either. Constipation or sitting on the toilet too long can be major culprits (another reason to put the damn phone away when you're pooping). I had a patient whose fissure developed when she tore during a routine colonoscopy to remove a benign growth. Sometimes it seems like everything and anything can cause a fissure. They're one of the most common anal ailments in the general population.

Acute fissures will generally go away on their own or with a little help from the topical creams and lotions I already mentioned. When fissures are chronic, it generally means something is keeping the skin from stretching as much as it needs to accommodate whatever it is you're using for anal play. The limiting factor could be the muscle, which won't dilate properly even though the skin has the capacity to stretch, or it could be the skin itself doesn't have the requisite elasticity even though the muscle below is capable of relaxing and stretching enough to bottom successfully.

A thorough sexual history will usually tell a doctor definitively whether a fissure is acute or chronic, but we can also find out by using an anoscope to look inside the anal canal. If we see a lot of scar tissue—especially in the front or back of the anus, the two weakest spots—that indicates a chronic fissure. Scar tissue is weak and tears easily under the pressure of defecation and anal play. But sometimes a patient complaining of anal pain will see multiple doctors who swear they can't see anything wrong, even though the sexual history makes it pretty clear a fissure is present. Often, these people are suffering from "phantom" fissures, rips in the skin that only appear during anal intercourse. They're not fake, just impossible to see during ordinary anal exams. Sometimes I'll just ask my patient to have sex or dilate before coming to their appointment, and then I'll take a look with the anoscope in the office. If we still don't see anything, I'll book them for the operating room, where while they're sedated I can dilate them far beyond what their pain threshold will currently allow them, to the extent necessary for me to see where the restrictive points are located and how the skin and muscle respond.

### Treatment Options

There are three levels of treatment for fissures, depending on their severity and chronicity: things you can do on your own (creams, lotions, suppositories and time), physical therapy and/or anal

Botox, and surgery. Determining which treatment to start with hinges not only on an assessment of the injury, but an assessment of what a patient is ready for. Many people are exhausted from trying to find answers, and agree to surgery right away if it means they can finally be rid of their pain. But many fear surgery and want to start slow, and I let them, even when I can see that the fissure can't be fixed without surgery. It's important to meet people where they are.

**Prescription-level anal fissure creams or lotions:** There are multiple brands doctors might recommend, many containing blood pressure medicine and nitroglycerin formulated for topical use, as they have been shown to help increase blood flow to the fissure. Extra blood flow promotes healing while helping relax the muscles in the area. Particularly helpful are compound lotions, usually formulated in specialty pharmacies. The compound I prefer combines diltiazem, a blood pressure medicine; lidocaine, a numbing medicine; and a topical steroid called Proctozone 2.5%. I tell my patients to dip their Calmol-4 suppositories into this compound medicine and insert them into their rectum twice per day, thus relaxing the muscles and bringing more blood to the area so that it heals faster.

**Botox:** We discussed in chapter 5 how well Botox can work to relax the muscles of the anus when the six-week dilation protocol is proving to be harder or taking longer than one might hope. It's also a game changer when it comes to treating fissures. When the body feels fear or pain, as it would with any kind of fissure, its inclination is to tighten up. In many people, their clenched muscles counteract the softening and soothing effects of the creams, ointments, and suppositories suggested above, preventing them from helping the ass heal. I almost always inject the Botox into the internal sphincter, but sometimes I'll also inject it into the fissure line. Adding Botox to the treatments decreases the pressure on the muscle and allows acute fissures to stay pliable and loose, which encourages the wound to heal correctly, which then allows patients to successfully dilate and enjoy sex. It's a five-minute, painless in-office procedure, similar in scope to getting Novocaine before dental work. There's no need for anesthesia. It takes about a week for the Botox to start working, and the effects last about three months. Most people need two-to-three rounds of Botox, in conjunction with dilation, stretching exercises, toys, and maybe gentle sex, to keep the muscle from snapping back to its original tight state.

For some people with an Anus Mediocris or Nope-us, stretching and dilating alone simply won't do the trick. Their muscles are like thick rubber bands that when stretched every day can get markedly looser, but can only go so far. Botox alone won't help, either. It can only relax the muscle; it can't increase its stretching capability. It's the combination of Botox plus dilation over time that relaxes and trains the muscle enough to stay pliable and open so people can achieve their goals.

Incidentally, Botox is also an excellent, safe, and longer-lasting alternative for anyone who regularly resorts to using amyl nitrite (poppers) and other drugs to help them relax before sex[1] (though if that's you, my hope is that after reading this book, you'll ditch those because you now know protocols and techniques to help you open up easily).

**Valium suppositories:** For anyone uncomfortable with needles or who doesn't need something as strong as a paralytic like

Botox, I offer diazepam suppositories. In pill form, diazepam is sold under the brand name Valium. Yep, "Mother's little helpers" are still around to help take the edge off, but in a completely different form than the depressed suburban housewives of the 1960s or the Rolling Stones, who sang about their plight, could have ever imagined. It's great for the patient who has enjoyed some dilation or sexual success yet needs a little more help stretching the muscles and skin to be able to get where they want to be. I also prescribe these suppositories to people suffering from anal fissures because they not only help relax the muscle, but also help calm the mind. Pain can take people on an emotional roller coaster. One day they feel better; the next day they try to bottom or just take an uneventful shit and realize they're not. The pain and uncertainty can ramp up people's anxiety and make it hard for them to relax, which works against their ability to heal.

**Physical therapy:** If possible, making an appointment with a physical therapist is not only helpful when you need a little extra guidance with the six-week dilation protocol, but the controlled environment and careful observation inherent in pelvic floor work can also help identify any specific issues that could be keeping the muscle and skin from healing. As we've also mentioned, a specially trained physical therapist can also observe when the problem isn't purely physical, but of a psychosexual or even neural nature.

If you don't have access to a physical therapist in your area, along with OTC medications and care that soothes and heals, careful dilation will be your best alternative to help give an acute fissure time to heal while keeping the muscles and skin strong and pliable. It's hugely beneficial to come back to your Booty

Camp protocol (page 77) with a new understanding of your body, keeping in mind what you've learned to prevent injury from reoccurring.

**Surgery:** I had a patient whose ass split after taking a larger-than-usual dick, and whose doctor performed a lateral sphincterotomy, which cuts the muscle to help it relax so the fissure can heal, to stop the constant bleeding every time he went to the bathroom. Yet the pain never let up. Bottoming was out of the question. Years later, when this suffering patient found me and I was able to take a look at his ass, I discovered that not only had the surgery done nothing to ease the muscle pressure in the anus, and not only was the initial fissure still present, but additional tissue had actually grown over it. When there's an underlying problem, such as excess scar tissue left over from an old injury, no matter how much dilation or Botox we try, we're not going to be able to get your butt to perform the way you want. Chronic anal injuries and problems can only be solved with surgery. This case was a classic example of how a medical practitioner's education and mindset affects the course of treatment. A lateral sphincterotomy may be warranted when you've tried everything else, when Botox works but only temporarily before the injury recurs, and when you've confirmed with a full manometry evaluation that the restrictive issue is indeed muscle tightness.

But this patient's doctor hadn't done any of that. He'd noted a fissure and extra scarring, but as is often the case in doctors who haven't made it a point to understand the bottoming community, he probably assumed that the only cause for such a condition would be that the muscle surrounding the injury was too tight to allow it to heal. He didn't think about how the friction of sex could cause that scar to repeatedly tear, probably because in his mind, that hole is exit-only. In fact, this patient's muscles weren't ever that tight. The entire problem was weak scar tissue, which cutting into muscle won't resolve. For cases like these—chronic scarring, extra tissue, maybe a gland causing a restriction—a fissurectomy, in which the damaged skin around the cut is removed, would be appropriate and effective. In fact, I can count on one hand how many times over the last twelve years I've ultimately had to cut into the anal muscle to resolve a patient's issues. I reserve them for people who've never successfully been able to take dick, who have developed significant scar tissue, or who regularly tear and can't relax in spite of multiple Botox treatments (most frequently body builders whose muscles are so overdeveloped nothing else is going to let them bottom the way they want to).

In general, however, fissurectomies are all that's needed, with simultaneous Botox treatments to help reset the pelvic floor, which has reflexively tightened up only in response to the pain of the fissure. I've seen many sphincterotomies performed in the wrong part of the ass or done in such a way as to cause excessive looseness, and it's doubly disturbing because in general the procedure didn't even need to be done in the first place. We need to look at all possible culprits—muscle, skin, *and* scar, not just the muscle, which is where most doctors focus.

## Hemorrhoids

You'll recall that there are two types of hemorrhoids, the veins designed to act as protective airbags in your ass—internal and external. The internal ones lie just above the dentate line of the anal canal (3–4 cm inside the asshole). While they can tear, bleed, and cause inflammation and swelling, they don't cause much pain. External symptomatic hemorrhoids, on the other hand, can hurt like hell, with additional symptoms that include swelling, itching, tightness, and bleeding. Most symptomatic hemorrhoids heal on their own with the help of the over-the-counter remedies we explored on page 217: soothing Epsom salt baths, Preparation-H cream, fiber supplements, and stool softeners. It also helps to use toilet paper as little as possible, more patting instead of wiping, foregoing wiping altogether in favor of a bidet—or even the shower when possible is even better. Please eliminate the use of baby wipes or medicated pads altogether.

When hemorrhoids impact a patient's quality of life, or repeatedly reoccur and hamper their ability to bottom or defecate without pain, we need to investigate why. Is it bad diet causing constipation? Is it crappy shitting technique? Is it too many squats at the gym? Is it a genetic issue? If the endgame is to enjoy anal sex, knowing the source of the problem is key. A doctor will be able to offer prescription-strength medical options to ease the symptoms, and guidance to help figure out what's causing the issue.

### Treatment Options

**Prescription-Strength Creams or Suppositories:** My patients with symptomatic hemorrhoids respond very well to the steroid Proctozone 2.5%. It comes in multiple forms: a suppository and foam for internal hemorrhoids as well as a cream for internal and external hemorrhoids. Sometimes it's combined with lidocaine for the numbing benefits.

**Botox:** If the hemorrhoid calms down but the muscles around it are still tight, it's likely the tightness is causing the hemorrhoid, not the other way around. Injecting Botox into the muscle surrounding the hemorrhoid can do a lot to decrease the pressure bearing down on the vein while simultaneously treating the hemorrhoid itself with OTC creams and ointments. I frequently use Botox as a preventative measure, too, to keep the hemorrhoid from flaring up again, and recommend dilation and physical therapy to address the underlying issue.

**Surgery:** If we've exhausted all these options and the hemorrhoid is still bothersome or causing additional symptoms, surgery is sometimes warranted. These are the most common surgical options:

**Cauterization:** Using an electric probe, a laser beam, or an infrared light, physicians can burn the hemorrhoid, causing it to close off and shrink. There is also chemical cauterization, which uses high doses of alcohol to destroy the hemorrhoid. I don't find cauterization to be particularly fruitful for bottoming patients except in cases where the hemorrhoid isn't that bad.

**Rubber band ligation:** This in-office technique is appropriate for small-to-medium size internal hemorrhoids, but not external ones at all. It involves using a special instrument to wrap a tiny rubber band around the base of the hemorrhoid, shutting off its blood supply and causing it to fall off within a week. The procedure can work great, but if you use ligation on someone whose hemorrhoids are actually being caused by extra tight muscles, the postsurgical pain and scarring can cause the muscle to tighten up even more, making the problem worse. You can imagine how much patients suffer when doctors often do as many as three ligations at once without addressing the muscle tightness that caused the flare in the first place. It's disastrous for people who want to bottom.

For patients who are able to engage sexually but who have a hemorrhoid that continually bleeds, if there's no underlying muscle tightness, cauterization or ligation can work well. In cases where tightness plays a role in the hemorrhoid flare-up, I'll start by administering Botox, and then do one ligation at a time so that we can see how the body responds and whether more ligations are actually necessary, or if the reset musculature allows the other hemorrhoids to permanently heal.

**Hemorrhoidectomy:** This procedure, which completely removes the hemorrhoids, is most appropriate for large internal hemorrhoids, uncomfortable external hemorrhoids, thrombotic hemorrhoids (which occur when a blood clot blocks blood flow, causing a bulge), or mild hemorrhoids that have resolved but left behind large amounts of excess skin (skin tags).

Most proctologists who aren't aware of or familiar with the needs of the anal community will treat everyone's asshole the same—same stitchwork, same protocols. So it's critical that when choosing a surgeon, you discuss and make sure they understand and respect your anal sex goals, needs, and desires, and know how to adjust their surgical technique accordingly. Depending on where the hemorrhoid is located, they can adjust the stitches to be a little tighter in someone who feels they're too loose, or leave room for the skin to heal with a lot more stretch, especially if they're working on someone who likes to take fists or especially large toys. They can also decide to only close the internal portion of the hemorrhoid, to prevent infection, but not the external portion, so that the skin has more room to stretch.

Recovery for either fissure or hemorrhoid surgery follows a similar trajectory. The first three to five days aren't much fun, despite the narcotic pain relievers you'll be prescribed. You'll be able to move around, but you'll be aware that something was done to your ass. (I'm told most of my surgical patients don't like me very much and curse me a lot during this phase.) You'll quickly transition from narcotics to NSAIDS, but still, for about two weeks after that, shitting will be uncomfortable. You can mitigate that discomfort with all the OTC treatments we've already discussed—Epsom salt baths, lotions, creams, and suppositories. You'll likely be able to go back to the gym in about five to seven days post-surgery, though you'll want to limit your leg work and squats. It's important to get back to your normal routine so your body heals to match your lifestyle.

Topping and jerking off will also be uncomfortable for about a week or two, and then that will start to feel normal again. Patients should see their doctors a month post-surgery to make sure everything is healing properly, at which point they should apply a chemical called silver nitrate into the scar to encourage wound healing and strengthening. This is an important step for people who want to bottom. Initial scars are very weak; silver nitrate helps get them into gladiator fighting form. At the two-month mark you'll be evaluated again, inspecting both inside and outside the anus, and then if all looks good, you can start your dilation training again, beginning all the way at the beginning with the smallest size in your kit. Most people are back to their regular sexual activities, including anal, within three months of surgery. The majority also get another round of in-office anal Botox to continue the positive trajectory. Recovery isn't much fun, but it's bearable when you keep your eye on the endgame.

## Skin Tags

Skin tags, which are extra folds of skin, can be side effects of injuries, such as hemorrhoids that get stretched out, or fissures in which the surrounding skin doesn't heal. Not all anal surgeons are concerned with ass aesthetics nor perceive a need to remove skin tags, which is why I have people from all over the world come to me after they've had an anal surgical procedure, asking me to go back in and remove the excess skin that has formed at or around the site. But even without injuries or surgery, the friction of anal sex can be enough to cause them to develop, or over time enlarge a previously small one to the extent that it hinders sex and makes it uncomfortable.

By themselves skin tags don't hurt, and some people love theirs, or their partners find them sexy. But others find they cause discomfort during sex, defecation, wiping, or even when wearing a thong. They might also just find them unsightly or know that their partners do, which makes them self-conscious in bed. Many anal surgeons dismiss the idea of removing them because they're harmless, but those of us who know and love the bottoming community understand that when a patient says their skin tags have gotta go, they gotta go.

Once again, your surgeon can choose to close things up good and tight or leave a little room for expansion depending on where the skin tags are located and your desires. Regardless, when the surgery is done, you should be left with a beautifully healed flat, flush tushhole.

Over time, some skin tags may resolve on their own, helped along by sitz baths (Epsom salt baths sold with a basin you can use if you don't have a tub) and Proctozone 2.5%, but in general, it takes surgery to get rid of them, either by cauterizing or excising them. If they're caused by something internal such as a fissure or hemorrhoids that need to go, the tags can be removed at the same time.

## Anal Gland Abscesses and Fistulas

Sometimes, the glands that line the anal canal and secrete mucus to lubricate our stools as we defecate can become clogged and infected with excrement, bacteria, semen, or oil and other skin debris, and form deep pockets full of pus called abscesses. The condition can be caused by sex, aggressive enema use, irritable bowel disease (IBD), and some STIs like herpes, HIV, chlamydia, and syphilis (which we'll discuss at length in the next chapter). But most of the time, it's a consequence of an infection. Abscesses can be extremely painful, especially when you sit down, during bowel movements and for people who bottom, who often report a burning sensation during receptive anal sex. In addition to pain, symptoms can include mucous discharge, bleeding, swelling, and constipation. Many people confuse hemorrhoids with abscesses. Pay close attention to your symptoms—if they're not improving, or there's worsening redness, or an increase in pain, it's typically not a hemorrhoid.

Abscesses sometimes heal on their own, but most of the time they need to be drained by a physician. It's a simple procedure after which the wound is generally left open to heal on its own, not even requiring stitches. The procedure is followed with antibiotics and tests to rule out an STI. And then we wait and observe. There are two reasons for that. The first is that frequently, my patient is in so much pain when they come to me, I can't do a thorough internal evaluation to see what might be obstructing the gland to cause the abscess. We have to drain it first to ease the pain. Then when my patient returns in four to six weeks for their follow-up appointment, I can take a look inside to see if any other conditions need to be treated to ensure the abscess doesn't recur. The second reason we need to watch and wait is that there's about a 50 percent chance that the drained abscess will develop into a fistula.

Fistulas occur when the infection from an abscess tunnels from the infection site into the soft tissue and muscle of the butt to eventually exit through the skin near the anus. From the outside, fistulas can look like pimples. A common symptom is a constant feeling of wetness from pus drainage. Symptoms can also include a hardening or swelling along the tunnel tract. Fortunately, fistulas aren't particularly painful, though they still suck.

There are two types of fistulas, simple and complex. If it's determined that a fistula is simple, meaning it doesn't have multiple tracts and doesn't compromise thirty percent or more of the

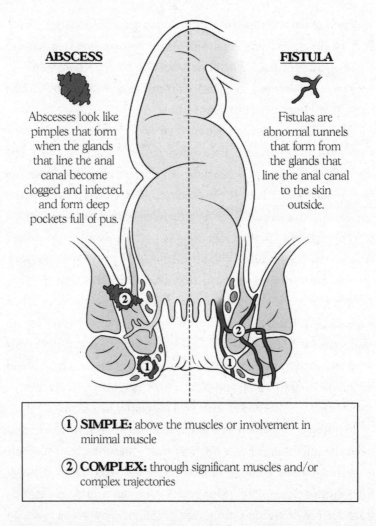

## ABSCESS

Abscesses look like pimples that form when the glands that line the anal canal become clogged and infected, and form deep pockets full of pus.

## FISTULA

Fistulas are abnormal tunnels that form from the glands that line the anal canal to the skin outside.

(1) **SIMPLE:** above the muscles or involvement in minimal muscle

(2) **COMPLEX:** through significant muscles and/or complex trajectories

external anal sphincter, a trained physician can simply open the tunnel to drain and let it heal on its own. Simple fistulas have low reoccurrence and complication rates. A complex fistula—one that affects thirty percent or more of the external sphincter, or has multiple tracts (which can indicate long-term inflammation or infection from inflammatory bowel diseases such as Crohn's disease or ulcerative colitis) needs a different surgical approach. There are multiple options (fistulas caused by IBD generally require a combination of medical and surgical treatments) but because fistula surgery success rates are highly dependent on the fistula's severity and location, I always try to choose the procedure that, should it fail, will fail in such a way as to leave the patient with a simple fistula or an improved position, which I can then return to easily address later, at which point it can heal. As always, it's critical for patients to work with surgeons who understand and respect their sexual desires, as some have been known to remove too much muscle, or not enough, and in these types of surgeries there are varying risks of incontinence and/or other complications.

## Scarring

Something that's almost always present and that I'm always looking for during an anal examination is scar tissue, both innate—the kind that forms over a natural cut or tear—and postsurgical, such as what would form after getting a hemorrhoid removed. Some people have a higher propensity to scar than others, but any scar tissue can potentially restrict the skin's capacity to stretch. Scars are some of the primary obstructions to successful bottoming. When a tear or abscess forms, and especially after a surgical procedure, someone who's been happily and easily enjoying anal sex for years can suddenly find themselves unable to receive. They can also become literal tight-asses, their poops narrowed to the size of a pencil because the accordions in their anal canal can't stretch wide enough to accommodate a normal-size bowel movement anymore.

These patients have generally been assured their anal injuries are healed, yet their pain or discomfort never lets up. Usually it's because while the original procedure was technically a success—the fissure is closed; the abscess or fistula is drained—the surgeon didn't consider the sexual nature of the bottoming community and didn't prescribe appropriate postoperative protocols that encourage the muscles and skin to stretch while healing. You don't realize how often you use your ass until you have a cut in there that refuses to heal. Sometimes the scar itself can get infected from collecting bits of excrement and mucus as it repeatedly builds and tears. It's a disaster for a bottom's sex life. I had one client who'd once been able to take so much dick his ass could have been, in his words, "bionic." Then one day out of the blue, he felt pain and bled every time he tried to bottom. It turned out he'd developed a fissure that created such restrictive scarring, he couldn't receive. By the time he came to me, four—FOUR!—surgeons later, his pain was so great he'd been celibate for three years.

With the right provider and all necessary topical, medical, and therapeutic treatments in place, it is possible to replace bad scar tissue with good scar tissue so that it's strong, pliable, and capable of stretching enough to reach the bottoming joys you desire. And even if we can't do that, there are surgical approaches that can tackle the scar once and for all. I had a patient from France who had multiple surgeries for hemorrhoids there that left him with significant scarring and limitations. He was suicidal. I worked on his scar twice to give more room, reshape and get him back to the bottoming game. Scarring is restrictive and limiting, but not the end-all.

## Rectal Prolapse and Looseness

Rectal prolapse occurs when the rectum partially or completely protrudes outside the ass. It's pretty rare. More commonly, swollen hemorrhoids bulge outside the anus, and these can be mistaken for rectal prolapse. Hemorrhoids, however, tend to be located along the sides of the anus and when they protrude, the folds are radial, like parallel lines. Rectal prolapse, however, involves tissue coming from deeper within the anal canal, and appears more circular. It generally happens when the suspensory ligaments that keep the rectum in place become too elastic, stretched either through the repeated push and pull of sex, or from pushing due to severe constipation. While it can be a side effect of fisting or taking large toys, size isn't everything. I've seen patients who take only ordinary dick and small toys yet suffered a prolapse because something was inserted at a bad angle, and I've had patients who would happily take Hercules, and everything would stay in place because they work at keeping those muscles strong and tight between sexual encounters.

Not everyone races to the doctor when they notice a prolapse—some people love the way it looks or feels, and even push it out to get a desired "rosebud" effect. In its less severe stages, the prolapse can be pushed back in and managed at home or through special exercise and therapy, such as Kegels, squats, and working with toys. In my office we have an Emsella chair, a specially designed chair that uses electromagnetic energy to stimulate and contract all the pelvic muscles, not just the ones controllable with Kegels. This noninvasive treatment can help increase contractility—the measure of tightness in the anus—by 20 percent, great news for people with early-stage rectal prolapse or even looseness. Eventually, however, repeated prolapse can become obstructive and interfere with everyday living, become uncomfortable or embarrassing, and, as it worsens, the risks of constipation and fecal incontinence rise. For these patients, surgery is the only option.

I'm seeing an uptick in younger people with rectal prolapse as fisting becomes more commonly depicted in porn and goes mainstream. Young muscles aren't always fully developed, which can be an advantage when they're asked to accommodate something large like fists and big toys, but eventually, those muscles are going to loosen. I love the fisting community. It's tight (ba-dum-bum), responsible, and it takes care of itself. Like dilation and ordinary anal sex, fisting successfully requires patience and training, and there are many in that population dedicated to helping people play safely. If fisting and big toys are your thing, learn proper squatting technique and practice pelvic floor work to counteract muscular looseness, for sure, but also seek out the advice and guidance of people with experience so you can train properly and avoid the downsides. In addition, I'd highly recommend yearly or every-other-year anal manometry tests to help keep track of your butt's muscle strength and condition. It allows you to map how your muscles change from year to year, allowing your doctor to know if Emsella treatments or pelvic floor therapy might be necessary to prevent looseness, and help you stay healthy.

———

Anal injuries and problems happen to everyone, not just those of us privy to the joys of anal play. The key to avoiding them as much as possible is education, self-awareness, and taking preventative steps, and addressing issues early, before they can become chronic. After reading this chapter, you should not only have a better awareness of what these symptoms can look and feel like, but also your options for resolving them. It's also a reminder that to get the proper treatment, you have to find a doctor who not only wants to understand the current problem, but also what your experience was before the problem occurred, and what end result you're hoping for once the problem has been fixed. If your doctor isn't asking you the questions that will tell them that, they're not the right practitioner for you. The sex life you want is yours for the taking, especially when you empower yourself by being your own advocate.

## CHAPTER 10

# The Truth About STIs

I had a client who sought help for a tear that wouldn't heal. He had visited multiple doctors, including a colorectal surgeon, who all tested his blood for STIs—negative—and sent him home with topical creams that did nothing for him. After many months, he found me. In addition to a regular exam at which I looked into the anal canal, I conducted a comprehensive STI screen, drawing blood but also getting a urine test and two oral swabs, one for chlamydia and gonorrhea, the other for herpes. Sure enough, the patient tested positive for chlamydia. As soon as he started treatment for the STI, the tear healed, and his pain stopped for good.

Any of the symptoms we covered in the last chapter—bleeding, pain, itching, soreness, and especially mucus or discharge—could be signs of undiagnosed bacterial or viral STIs, which can feed off irritated, bleeding, and inflamed wounds and prevent them from healing. In fact, the lurking STI could have been why your butt was susceptible to the injury or condition that caused the symptoms in the first place. If you experience these symptoms and there's any chance it could be an STI, you need to pay a visit to the doctor to get tested, because none of these issues will resolve without treating the infection first.

It's not a small possibility. With few exceptions, to be sexually active is to be at risk for STIs. The 2021 CDC analysis of the incidence and prevalence of STIs in the United States reported that 20 percent of the population was infected with an STI at any given time in 2018. That's about one in five.[1] And while the risk of HIV has greatly decreased as more and more people have started taking Pre-exposure prophylaxis (PrEP), according to the CDC, that number represents only about *one-quarter* of those for whom a prescription is recommended,[2] and PrEP doesn't prevent against other common STIs like syphilis, chlamydia, and gonorrhea, or sexually transmitted viruses like herpes and hepatitis B[3]. Contrary to bigoted stereotypes, the increased rates of STIs aren't solely manifesting in the MSM community—almost half of the 26 million new cases of STIs per year in the United States are found in young people ages fifteen to twenty-four.[4] With numbers like that, unless you require your partner(s) to use a condom each and every time you bottom, you're at significant risk.

Despite their ubiquity, STIs are not something to take casually. When left untreated, many can have serious health repercussions, such as neurological and cardiovascular disease[5], increased rates of various types of cancers, and a heightened risk of acquiring more STIs and/or HIV in all populations[6] including those taking pre-exposure prophylactics (PrEP). Many can also affect people's genitalia and reproductive organs, compromising fertility and complicating conception, pregnancy, and childbirth, as well as potentially infecting an unborn baby in people AFAB, even when the STI was contracted before the baby was conceived.

The number of new STI cases documented in 2018 cost the U.S. healthcare system $16B in lifetime medical costs.[7]

Fun stuff, right? I know that talking about STIs feels like a total downer and that you'd much rather I continue to feed you juicy tips that will add oomph to your orgasms and make your partners swoon, and I will—just wait until we get to the booty beauty tips in the next chapter! But I promise you that although the subject matter in this chapter is serious, it isn't all doom and gloom. Once again, you're not in a high school sex ed class where the curriculum's main goal is to scare the shit out of you and keep you from having sex. With early diagnosis and treatment, several of the most common STIs can be cured, all can be managed, and their effects minimized if not eradicated. Best of all, as of this writing, not one is a death sentence.

Despite not being something to take casually, STIs aren't anything to be ashamed or embarrassed about. The fact is, there's a good chance more than one person you know, including straight, non-anal-engaging ones, are infected but asymptomatic. No one catches these things because they're degenerates or sluts; they're just one of the possible consequences of being sexually active, just like pregnancy and UTIs in people AFAB, or fissures and hemorrhoids in people who love anal sex. And just like pregnancy, UTIs, and anal injuries, the more you know about what causes them and the preventative measures you can take to avoid them, the less risk you run of ever having to deal with them. But even when we take every precaution, shit happens, and I want you to know what to do. The more openly and honestly we discuss STIs, the faster we can break their harmful stigma and protect ourselves and each other. Besides, just because they won't kill you doesn't mean they can't make you damn uncomfortable and put a damper on your sex life. For this reason alone it's worth minimizing your risk of infection!

> May we never forget all those we lost to the AIDS epidemic of the 1980s and '90s, nor stop honoring the activists who fought to raise awareness about the disease, demanded the government and medical community dedicate funds for research and developing treatments, and who insisted that the millions of HIV carriers and AIDS patients in the world be treated with dignity and respect.

I'm not a primary care doctor nor an infectious disease specialist, but I talk to everyone who comes into my office about how to curtail STI exposure. If I see it, I treat it. I'll also ask you how you think you got it, not because I want to judge, but because I want to help you mitigate risk. Do you think you got it through a random hookup? Did your partner cheat? Do you and your partner stay healthy when it's just the two of you, but bring something home every time you attend sex parties? If so, we need to talk about what preventative and protective measures you could adopt. When you analyze your behavior and take steps to lower your risk of catching an STI, it helps lower the risk for the entire community.

I don't care what decisions you make; I just want you to be informed when you make them so you can enjoy worry-free sex. With that goal in mind, we're going to run through the most common STIs you're likely to come across—bacterial, viral, and parasitic—their available treatments, and preventative care. That means this chapter is going to be a bit more science-y and medical than most of the other ones in this book. Just think of this chapter as probiotic and fiber for your brain, bulking up your sexual health knowledge and protecting you so you can keep having anal sex as frequently and safely as you please.

I'm going to focus on the anal manifestations of these infections because that's my area of expertise and the focus of this book, but it's important to note that some STIs can present symptoms on genitalia, orally, or be asymptomatic. Just because you contract an infection anally doesn't mean it won't migrate or manifest elsewhere. Just because you don't see any symptoms doesn't mean you don't have an STI. In addition, more than one thing can be true simultaneously. You could have a microtear causing you a little blood and pain, *and* have contracted an STI whose symptoms are—you guessed it—a little blood and pain.

If you think you may have been exposed, I urge you to seek out additional information on these infections from reputable sources such as the CDC, the WHO, Planned Parenthood, and your primary doctor. It's also imperative that you notify your partners or fuck buddies—anyone with whom you come into sexual contact—and do your part to help curtail community spread. We're all in this together.

---

## If You Learn Nothing Else...

I know that not all of you are going to read this chapter, no matter how much I wish you would. I've said it before and I'll say it again: You are your own best health advocate, and I promise that knowing the not-so-sexy stuff will ultimately make your sex life that much hotter and more carefree. That said, if you do plan to skip, please know that these symptoms *always* require medical attention:

- Worsening anal pain
- Worsening bleeding with mucous and discharge
- Fever, chills, and generalized malaise and fatigue within a few days or weeks of a sexual encounter

If you're experiencing these symptoms, or recently had an unprotected (i.e., no condoms) sexual encounter with someone who is, call your healthcare provider or go to your nearest Planned Parenthood or community center for STI testing. Understand, however, that STI symptoms can develop weeks, months, or years after infection, or even never at all, which is why it truly is in your best interest to educate yourself now.

## BACTERIAL AND VIRAL STIS

The most common pain-in-the-ass infections are caused by bacteria or viruses. Bacteria are living organisms that don't need a host to survive, though we have billions living in and on our bodies, including in the gut and anus, where, as we discussed in our conversations about diet and douching (see chapters 6 and 7), they absorb nutrients and keep the growth of bad bacteria in check, keeping our bodies healthy and functioning smoothly. Viruses, on the other hand, need a host to reproduce and survive. Regardless, they're both pains in the ass. Infections arise when harmful bacteria proliferate, or a virus infiltrates our healthy cells. It can be hard to know based on symptoms alone whether an infection is bacterial or viral, since symptoms can be similar. When you know what to look for, however, some signs can give you a clue that can speed diagnosis and inform your doctor's treatment plan, especially since some of these infections require long-term management.

## Bacterial STIs

I'm going to start with the good news right up front: bacterial STIs are not only treatable, they're also curable, sometimes with a single dose of an antibiotic. Like the carriers of many STIs, however, a lot of people walk around not knowing they've been infected, and if left untreated, bacterial STIs can have serious consequences down the line. So it's worth it to know the signs and best preventative measures.

### *Gonorrhea and Chlamydia*

**SYMPTOMS**

The symptoms for these two common STIs are similar, though some people, especially those who are AFAB, never exhibit symptoms. Both can cause white, yellow, or green discharge from the anus, bleeding from the rectum during defecation, and constipation due to swelling and pain.

**DIAGNOSIS**

Swabbing the affected area and taking urine samples are the general protocol for testing for and diagnosing both infections. Note that there are separate tests for oral, anal, and genital chlamydia and gonorrhea. A negative test for one type doesn't preclude a positive test for another. If you think you're at risk, get tested for everything.

## TREATMENT

Gonorrhea and chlamydia are often treated with common antibiotics like doxycycline or ceftriaxone IM injection, ranging from a 7–21-day treatment (depending on how complicated the infection is), a shot in the ass, or a combination of both. In especially severe or delayed cases, I recommend serial reswabbing to make sure the infection is actually gone.

## Syphilis

### SYMPTOMS

Syphilis presents with small, painless sores called chancres on the genitals or mouth, indicating where the infection entered the body. They ooze fluid, but they can often go unnoticed if they're not easily visible. Even once the chancres heal, between one to five weeks after infection, at this stage syphilis is highly contagious. If left untreated, it can travel through several stages, ranging in severity from rashes to muscle weakness, cognitive difficulties, and vision and hearing loss in the rare tertiary stage, which can occur decades after infection.

### DIAGNOSIS

Blood test or sample from an oozing sore. There are two tests: One to show you are acutely positive or have been exposed to syphilis, called RPR; and one called a titer, which measures antibodies in the blood to reveal whether this is a previous infection or an active one, and if active, how full-blown. It's important to find out where you stand. It can take a long time for the infection to reveal itself, and months to a year for results to get to normal range. This is why it's good to get an STI screening every three months (which is required for people already on PrEP)—you could get a negative result only because you tested too soon after contracting the illness. You could also remain asymptomatic for months, increasing the risk of you inadvertently passing it on to someone else. If you believe you could be at risk, it's important to keep testing to make sure your initial diagnosis isn't a false negative.

## TREATMENT

A single dose of penicillin cures all the early stages, and a few rounds of doses can cure the rare late stages of the disease. There are other treatments, too, including a 21-day course of doxycycline. Despite the effectiveness of treatment, just as it can take a long time for the illness to reveal itself in bloodwork, it can take up to a year for those blood test results to come back normal. Once you're asymptomatic and the antibody titer numbers measured in your blood keep decreasing, you're no longer considered infectious. However, treatment cannot reverse any damage that may have already occurred.

## PREVENTION

In some populations, such as MSM already taking PrEP, taking a single dose of the antibiotic doxycycline has been shown to dramatically lower the incidence of chlamydia, gonorrhea, and syphilis when taken within forty-eight hours of exposure[8] (and a preliminary study found that gargling with Listerine mouthwash could be an effective way to reduce the risk of oral gonorrhea in MSM[9]). Some people might be concerned that taking antibiotics without any evidence of infection could contribute to antibiotic resistance, undermining the effectiveness of current treatments. But actually, when compared to the 21-day course of antibiotics required to treat a full-blown infection, you wind up taking far fewer doses. In addition, this approach minimizes the chances of an asymptomatic person unknowingly spreading the infection to their partners. It's not just your ass on the line, it's the whole community's.

## Viral STIs

### Herpes

An extremely common STI is the herpes simplex virus (HSV). Carriers can often go their whole lives without knowing they're infected. It's treatable and manageable, but not curable. While some symptoms can be uncomfortable, the most painful aspect of herpes is the unnecessary stigma surrounding it.

#### SYMPTOMS

When symptoms do appear, they can be in the form of blisters, ulcers, or sores that eventually burst and crust over. Sometimes people describe feeling like they have thousands of paper cuts around their anus, and confuse them with the kind of irritation often caused by wet wipes. (It bears repeating—stay away from wet wipes!) There are two types of the virus. HSV-1—the type that can cause what we often call cold sores or fever blisters—is so common, it's estimated that between fifty to eighty percent of U.S. adults have it.[10] It's spread orally, and symptoms typically appear around the mouth, though they can also manifest on genitals. In my office, I tend to see a lot of anal cases of herpes type-1. Why? Rimming, of course. It's the best, but all that oral ass-pleasuring gives the virus ample opportunities to jump from mouth to butt.

HSV-2 is spread only through sexual contact, and causes genital blisters that burst and result in painful sores. Some people experience nerve pain. People with penises sometimes experience difficulty or pain while urinating, depending on where the blisters form, and both penis owners and people with vaginas might experience smelly discharge. With both types of herpes, patients often report an itching or burning sensation in the areas where the blisters will eventually erupt. Outbreaks can be triggered by illness (hence the name "cold sores"), stress, sun exposure and hormonal changes. Also, excess moisture. (Which means what? One more time for the people in the back: Stay away from wet wipes!)

### DIAGNOSIS

When blisters or sores are present, doctors can send a swab of fluid to a lab to determine which type of herpes is present. This test is most accurate within the first 48 hours of the symptoms appearing. After that, there's a good chance for a false negative. If there are no symptoms, your doctor can administer a blood test. Unfortunately, the test doesn't detect the virus, it detects antibodies, which proves that at some point your immune system mounted a defense against the virus. All this tells you is that at some point you were exposed to HSV-1 or HSV-2; it can't confirm an acute infection. It's shocking how many patients have come to me with sores, ulcerations, and pain—all classic symptoms of HSV-1 and -2—who've been prescribed multiple rounds of antibiotics that of course did nothing for them, yet were never swabbed for herpes. That said, I can't think of a time that I had a truly asymptomatic patient, even if they only had HSV-1. More likely, people have minor symptoms but ignore them, and thus remain undiagnosed for a long time until they come in for something else or a regular checkup. They'll mention they're itchy or that their ass burns a little when they wash it with soap and water. I'll do a swab, and the test will come back positive. We could curb the spread and reduce people's suffering by a lot if HSV swabbing was standard practice.

**TREATMENT**
Antiviral medications like valacyclovir (brand name Valtrex) and acyclovir (brand name Zovirax) are your best options for speeding up healing and reducing the reoccurrence of symptoms. Though it's expensive, if your insurance covers it, I like to suggest an additional topical antiviral acyclovir cream.

Important to know is that even when successfully treated and healed, genital herpes can still increase a carrier's risk of HIV infection.[11]

**PREVENTION**

If you're in a relationship with someone who has genital herpes, or you've experienced two or more infections, taking a daily preventative dose of valacyclovir can help ease the symptoms and reduce the frequency of repeated outbreaks.[12]

## *HPV*

Human papillomavirus (HPV) is the most common sexually transmitted infection in the United States, with roughly 13 million new cases per year.[13] Among MSM, reports show the prevalence of HPV ranges between about 60 percent in the general population, to up to 90 percent in MSM living with the HIV virus.[14] According to the CDC, at least four out of every five people AFAB will have at one point been infected with HPV.[15] Congratulations, there's a good chance you've gone viral even if you only have 46 social media followers!

Why are these numbers so high? The virus is extremely easy to transmit. Entering the body through a cut, abrasion, or small tear in the outer layer of your skin, it's most commonly transferred through intercourse and skin-to-skin or skin-to-mucosa contact. That means kissing, touching, oral sex, rimming, and fucking, both with a condom and raw. In other words, all the good stuff. It's easily spread even when the carrier is asymptomatic, which describes almost everybody. The majority of people infected with HPV never know they have it because their immune systems quickly clear up the infections. People come to me for all kinds of reasons. They know they have warts; they're having symptoms, but they don't know what's causing them; or they've had an anal Pap smear that needs further internal evaluation.

## SYMPTOMS

When symptoms do manifest, they could appear a few days after transmission, or a few years. Frequently, people discover they have HPV because of the appearance of genital warts, which can appear on or in the anus, genitals and the surrounding skin, the lining of the vagina, the cervix, the face, and/or the mouth and throat (your dentist should be checking for these during regular cleanings and checkups). The warts can look like a small bump or a group of bumps. Sometimes they take on a cauliflower shape. They can be raised or flat, gray or skin-colored, visible or almost invisible. The warts can feel like lumps or look like lesions, and while they aren't painful themselves, when large or plentiful enough the growths can cause friction or restriction, which can cause pain and even constipation. Many patients come to see me thinking they have skin tags, and are surprised and dismayed when instead we have to have a conversation about STIs.

Sometimes there are no external warts, and yet people experience itching, bleeding, or mucus discharge, and warts are found with an internal digital and anoscopic exam at the doctor's office. Some people may have no symptoms at all, but an abnormal Pap smear (a test that takes cell samples) comes back positive, which then requires an internal exam revealing the presence of asymptomatic anal warts. Many people, on their yearly examinations, routinely do an anoscopic exam to ensure anal health, and sometimes anal warts are present even though the Pap smear results come back normal. There's just no predictable pattern to how this STI manifests. But warts are really not that big of a deal. They're incredibly common, and if treated appropriately, short-lasting.

There are many permutations of HPV manifestation, but for the purposes of this book, we're going to keep things simple and just focus on what to do if you have warts, and the importance of early detection and management through yearly anal Pap smears, and internal and external evaluations.

## DIAGNOSIS

Many times warts present externally, so all a doctor has to do is take a look at your junk to offer a formal diagnosis of HPV. However, since warts can also grow internally, even above the dentate line, and can be tiny, your physician should also conduct an internal examination with a colposcope, which has a high power of magnification, so you can learn the extent of the problem. Even though most warts aren't cancerous or even dysplastic (showing changes that could lead to cancer), it's routine to biopsy the warts just to rule out the possibility that something could be forming. Treatment protocols will be determined by whether you present with external warts, internal warts, or a combination.

## TREATMENT

First things first: you gotta get rid of the warts. They can be pesky little fuckers that require multiple rounds of treatment. Sometimes patients will see a dermatologist, who of course treats the external warts, but they keep returning until the patient visits a physician who does an internal exam which reveals that, lo and behold, there are internal warts as well. You have to have an external and internal examination to know the correct course of treatment, but with proper management, warts can be eradicated.

You can remove mild to moderate cases of internal and external warts by freezing them off through cryosurgery or burning them off with a laser or, my preference, electrocautery. A mild case can be treated as an in-office procedure, whereas a more severe case may lend itself to procedures that require anesthesia. Internally, trichloroacetic acid can also be used to chemically burn off the warts. Creams like Imiquimod, Podophyllin, Podofilox, and Sinecatechins are good for getting rid of external warts, too. Sometimes these warts are hard to see, and often when I remove them externally, new ones will pop up right next to the removal site. Smearing these creams all over the external anal area can prevent that from happening and is the preferred removal method. (These creams are not to be used internally.) If they work, I'll put my patients on an extended dose for eight to sixteen weeks.

Do not ever try to use over-the-counter wart removal medications on genital warts! First, they can cause painful irritation and burns on the delicate genital skin. Second, it's not an easy-to-view location, and it's important you see a physician to get a confirmed diagnosis before applying any wart treatment. Finally, what you see on the outside of your ass may be just the tip of the iceberg; if there are internal lesions inside where you can't see them, it will be useless to try to treat the external warts.

---

Even when the warts are cleared, once infected with HPV, always infected with HPV. It's treatable, it can be managed and its impact minimized, but once you've got it, you've got it for life.

If I've removed anal warts, I see my patients in three months. If there are still no signs of warts, I'll see them again in six months, followed by regular annual exams. The key with anal wart management is aggressive follow-up.

## DYSPLASIA

Whether warts develop or not, multiple types of HPV strains can cause anal dysplasia, which is when cells around the anus transform into precancerous, abnormal cells that have a higher likelihood of multiplying and transitioning into cancer. It's estimated that 90 percent of anal cancer is caused by HPV.[16] The presence of warts is in no way indicative that you have anal dysplasia or cancer, however. Should your doctor find signs of dysplasia, even after removing any warts that might be present, you don't need to panic. Any number of things, such as hemorrhoids, skin tags, or scars, can cause a positive result even though there's no actual precancerous change.[17]

Dysplasia is detected through anal Pap smears, which take a sample of your anal cells, which are then sent to a pathologist. Typically, doctors take two swabs, especially during an initial evaluation. The first sample of cells will be tested to determine the specific strain of HPV, if present, and the second will be analyzed for precancerous or cancerous risk. Pap smear results note any changes in a cell and grade those changes on a scale of low-to-high risk.

If your Pap smear results are positive, your doctor may send you to a specialist to perform an HRA (high resolution anoscopy) with biopsy, which are actually multiple biopsies with special staining techniques, since you need to sample a range of tissue in the area. The results of those biopsies will determine what direction your treatment will take, with many options that are beyond the scope of this book. The immediate step is to eradicate the abnormal cells to prevent cancer from developing. Your doctor may use some of the procedures mentioned above for wart removal, or they might decide the tissue should be ablated, which means removing the top layer of cells, usually via cautery (heat) to allow healthy tissue to grow.

Sometimes doctors will find that anal cancer is present. The standard options for treatment are chemotherapy and radiation, which thankfully frequently achieve extremely effective results. You should have an open dialogue with your doctor and be informed of all the risk factors as you determine how aggressively and quickly to proceed. Ultimately, each case is unique and multifactorial, so you and your provider can determine the best course of action for you.

Anal Pap smears are incredibly valuable. Repeated, regularly scheduled anal Pap smears will allow your doctor to follow your HPV trajectory and make sure to catch any precursory signs of cancer long before they can develop into something serious. Key to getting an accurate diagnosis of HPV is finding a doctor that not only performs anal Pap smears, but performs them correctly. In a proper anal Pap smear, your provider will insert a swab that looks like a long Q-tip two or three inches into your anus to collect a sampling of cells from the surface. (From now on you'll probably never look at a real

Q-tip quite the same way again. Sorry about that.) When making your appointment, ask if your doctor uses a cervical brush or a Q-tip swab to take the samples. A cervical brush resembles and feels like a pipe cleaner, and is not only too abrasive for the anus, but in my experience frequently results in false positives. If they don't use or offer to use the Q-tip swab, find someone who will.

## PREVENTION

Aside from correct, consistent condom use (read: every time!), the best prevention against HPV is immunization. Approved in 2006 for pre-teens ages 11–12, the vaccine Gardasil protects against nine types of HPV, including the strains linked to genital warts and cancer. Since its approval in 2006, cases of the HPV types that cause cervical cancer have decreased by almost 90 percent in young people AFAB, rates of genital warts in all young people are down,[18] and the incidence of anal warts in young people AMAB up to the age of 24 are down by one-third.[19] This shit works!

The vaccine has since been approved for use in patients up to age 45, but I encourage all my patients no matter their ages to get vaccinated, although for older patients the cost is higher because it's out of pocket and at this time costs over $285.00 per shot.[20] Full protection requires three shots, though recently we've seen new data that one to two shots may also be effective.[21] In my practice I see reasons for older men to get it, as their relationships and sexual practices commonly change as they age, with avowed tops frequently becoming bottoms. The vaccine won't protect against any strains of HPV to which you may have already been exposed, but it can protect you from new strains. Anecdotally, I've seen a decrease in the reoccurrence of anal warts and an increase in the speed with which issues resolve.

And please, quit the butt wipes. Butt wipe use frequently correlates with external warts. HPV-positive people who've never had warts in their lives can start using wipes and, boom, see warts develop. People who don't yet have HPV and start using butt wipes don't realize they're irritating the skin and creating an entryway and fertile breeding ground for the infection. There's no way to prove which came first in these cases, but we do know that anybody who uses wipes either has a higher propensity of their known HPV to develop into anal warts, or they have a higher propensity to contract HPV due to increased inflammation.

## *HIV*

Entire books have been written on the human immunodeficiency virus (HIV) and the physical, emotional, and psychological toll the AIDS crisis of the 1970s, '80s, and '90s had on the LBTQ+ population, especially gay men. There was a time when this chapter would have been dominated by the topic of HIV and the specter of AIDS; a time when hooking up bareback was dancing with fire, practically a suicidal pact. It's a testament to how incredibly far we've come that I can devote about as much space to HIV as I did to anal warts. Because while there is still no cure for HIV, it can be managed with proper treatment. In fact, today's young people are the first generation able to think about this disease as just one of many manageable conditions humans learn to live with. The arrival of PrEP on the scene means HIV as an illness is a less urgent issue than the fact that so many people think that if they're on PrEP it's safe to forgo condoms, raising the risks of STIs. And the best way to honor the hundreds of thousands who didn't get to see this day is to live out and proud, to celebrate our sexuality, and to allow ourselves to freely give and receive the gifts of intimacy, passion, or just the satisfying thrill of a good hookup, all while taking proper precautions and educating ourselves so we can weigh and mitigate risk.

HIV is transmitted between adults through sexual contact and needle-sharing when injecting drugs. When left untreated in its late stages, HIV develops into acquired immune deficiency syndrome (AIDS). Forty percent of new cases are transmitted by people who don't know they have the virus.[22]

## SYMPTOMS

The earliest symptoms of HIV can start about two to four weeks after acquiring the virus, and might feel a lot like the flu, such as enlarged lymph nodes, sore throat, fever, chills, fatigue, and unexplained weight loss. Some people experience rashes and night sweats. These symptoms often go away within a week to a month, which is why so many people fail to realize they've been infected. Unfortunately, it's during that early period of time, when people are unaware they're carriers, that the risk of transmission to others is at its highest. This is why regular, frequent STI testing, as outlined later in this chapter, is so important, especially as many of the symptoms could easily be mistaken for signs of flu or COVID.

### DIAGNOSIS

If you suspect a recent exposure, within ten days to a month, a nucleic acid test (NAT) may be able to detect the virus in your bloodstream. However, most people won't get tested until they experience symptoms, at which point antibody or antigen blood tests, or even a finger stick, can be performed to check for HIV exposure. HIV and other STI testing are becoming increasingly available in all areas, meaning the new generation of anal players are very likely to take getting checked seriously.

### TREATMENT

**ART:** For HIV-positive patients, daily antiretroviral therapy (ART) can lower a carrier's viral load to undetectable levels, meaning there is so little virus in the blood it can't be measured in a lab. At undetectable levels, HIV is no longer infectious and can't be passed to HIV-negative partners. Today, HIV-positive people who consistently stick to their treatments can have the same life expectancy as those who are HIV-negative. It's no longer a death sentence. This development has been game-changing in lifting the stigma of being HIV-positive, to the point that people now include their status—especially U=U (undetectable means untransmittable)—in their dating profiles and hookup apps.

### PREVENTION

**PrEP:** This is one hell of a success story. Since its approval by the FDA in 2012, when taken consistently, the HIV prevention medication PrEP (pre-exposure prophylactic) has been shown to decrease the risk of getting HIV through sex by 99 percent, and through needle-sharing by as much as 74 percent.[23] PrEP is available in pill form or by injection. It's covered by most insurance plans and state Medicaid programs. For the uninsured, city and state clinics, hospitals and outpatient facilities, and even the makers of the drugs, will pay for or partially cover the cost of PrEP for eligible candidates.

Everyone who engages in anal should talk to their doctor about getting on PrEP. See the end of the chapter for dosage options.

**Condoms:** When used correctly (lots and lots of lube) and consistently—i.e., always—condoms alone reduce the risk of HIV to bottoms by 72 percent. For tops, it's 63 percent.[24] It's worth noting that as of 2020, only a quarter of the U.S. population for whom PrEP would be recommended take it,[25] so condoms are a really, really good idea.

## Intestinal Parasites

One testing protocol that should be standard in STI management, but unfortunately isn't, are stool studies. The anal community is prone to parasitic infections—in one controlled study, over 65 percent of a tested population tested positive for intestinal parasites[26]—yet people are rarely tested unless they present with the bloating, diarrhea, or other GI issues that are common symptoms. Meanwhile, parasitic STIs are frequently asymptomatic.

When they're not, though, they can be super uncomfortable. There are two in particular you should be aware of if you're having anal sex; and especially if you're into rimming, there are steps you can take to protect yourself.

### Giardia and Entamoeba histolytica

Giardia is a microscopic parasite that lives in the intestines and is passed out in feces. Once outside the body, it can sometimes survive for weeks or months. In the anal community, it's often spread via oral-anal contact, and contaminated toys are often the source of recurrent infections. It's the most frequently diagnosed intestinal parasitic disease in the United States and the world.[27]

Entamoeba histolytica is another microscopic parasite that lives in the intestines and is passed out through poop. It's spread when hands or toys that have touched contaminated feces are put in the mouth. It's also communicable through oral-anal contact.[28]

#### SYMPTOMS

Carriers of either of these parasites will usually remain asymptomatic, but when symptoms do present, they start one to three weeks after infection. Giardia frequently presents in the form of diarrhea, greasy stools, gas, and abdominal cramps.[29] Entamoeba histolytica can cause amebiasis, the symptoms of which are diarrhea, stomach pain, and stomach cramps. In severe cases, it can lead to amebic dysentery, which manifests as bloody stools, stomach pain, and fever. Rarely, the parasite can migrate to the liver and cause an abscess.[30]

## DIAGNOSIS

Rectal swabs (for rimmee) and oral swabs (for rimmer), as well as stool samples, often collected over the course of several days. Because stool sampling is not a routine test, you will probably have to ask your doctor to perform one. Request specifically that they test for both ova and parasites.

## TREATMENT

Both Giardia and Entamoeba histolytica can be treated with Metronidazole, an antibiotic, or other antiparasitic medications.[31] Depending on the strain isolated and the severity of amebiasis symptoms, patients may be prescribed two different types of antibiotics.[32]

## PREVENTION

Since Entamoeba histolytica and Giardia are especially easy to spread through rimming, if you're into analingus, or think it could be a possibility during a tryst, cleaning any area where a tongue might go before sex is a must. That does NOT mean you should douche, though you can. Rather, it means using gentle soap and water to clean the external anal region, along with the rim, the beginning of the anal canal, and anywhere even Kiss front man Gene Simmons's tongue could reach.

Wash your hands pre- and post-play. The same goes for anything that might be used for penetration, like sex toys, fingers, and other body parts. Afterward, rinse your mouth with an antiseptic mouthwash to kill off any potential bacteria, though do avoid brushing your teeth for at least an hour to prevent microtears, which facilitate STI transmission. In addition, a prophylactic regimen with the antibiotic Metronidazole has been shown to decrease Giardia rates of infection.

## HOW LONG AFTER MY STI SYMPTOMS ARE GONE BEFORE I CAN HAVE SEX AGAIN?

This is often the first and most urgent question I get after diagnosing someone with an STI. Refraining from sex during the first three to five days of treatment for any STI is key to make sure you're improving. Ideally, you'd refrain from sex until you're completely asymptomatic, and then go back to using toys, stretching, and dilating to make sure everything feels good and that your butt is ready to receive. For severe infections, it would be best to retest to make sure you're truly infection-free before engaging. That's not only in your partners' best interests, because you don't want to pass the infection to others, but also in your own, because if you go back to sexual activity before you're fully healed, you have a higher risk of recurrence.

## UNIVERSAL STI PREVENTION ADVICE

Unless you're in a strictly monogamous sexual relationship with someone who has no STIs, if you lick, suck, or fuck, take these steps to keep yourself and your community healthy and safe:

**Test, test, test.** Get tested every three months for STIs, symptoms or no symptoms. If you're having repeated STIs or attending sex parties, test every month. Regular, frequent testing is imperative, especially in an era when so many illnesses like COVID and flu have similar symptoms, to ensure the earliest treatment and prevent inadvertent spreading of infections, especially HIV. These exams should include bloodwork (making sure to check the usual STIs, along with kidney and liver function if you're on PrEP and/or Valtrex); an internal and external anal examination, checking specifically for anal warts and herpes, including an annual anal pap smear; and a urine test and swabs, both anal and oral, to test for chlamydia and gonorrhea. Though not routinely done, I also think it should be standard to conduct stool studies to check for parasites, and anal herpes swabs, because people often don't otherwise know they're infected.

Some labs will ask you to perform the swabs yourself. You should refuse. More often than not, patients asked to do their own swabs are uncomfortable with the process and don't insert the swab far enough. Too often, I meet patients who performed the test themselves and got inaccurate results, which just further delayed treatment. If your doctor won't do this or any of the other tests, find another physician who will.

Even if you get regularly tested but after an encounter you think there's the potential for you to have contracted an STI—if you had unprotected sex, or if the thought crosses your mind even once—go see a doctor or visit a sexual health clinic for a thorough screening.

**Get a yearly anal pap smear.** The same test that can be used to diagnose HPV is what can help you prevent anal cancer through early detection. Commit to getting a yearly annual exam. (People AFAB are probably thinking, goddamn, now I have to get *two* of these every year?) It will give you peace of mind and access to preventative healthcare, as your doctor will not only take a swab, but will be able to visually inspect the area to make sure everything looks healthy back there. Ideally, they would perform an inside and outside anoscopy.

**Use condoms.** Consistent use of condoms substantially reduces the risk of HPV transmission, especially in nonmonogamous people AMAB, and decreases the duration of infection in those who are high-risk. Condoms are especially effective when used in tandem with the HPV vaccine, and protect against strains the HPV vaccine doesn't cover.[33] Remember that condoms only prevent transmission in the areas they cover, as anywhere you have unprotected contact is a susceptible infection site. If you have an outbreak, refrain from sexual activity to help stop the spread until your symptoms subside. That includes steering clear of oral sex if you have a cold sore or feel one coming on, as that may be indicative of a herpes infection.

**Get vaccinated.** Get the HPV vaccine, even if you're older than 45 years. Bottoming always carries an increased risk of HPV transmission, regardless of the bottom's age.

**Talk to your doctor about PrEP.** There are now various forms of PrEP depending on what suits your needs. You can take a daily dose, a bi-monthly injection, or if you're in a somewhat committed relationship and know when you're going to have sex, you can try "on-demand" PrEP, also known as PrEP 2-1-1, which has you take two pills two to twenty-four hours before sex, one pill twenty-four hours after the first dose, and one pill twenty-four hours after the second dose. The option that works best for you will depend on your lifestyle and ability to remember a pill regimen.

**Play clean.** Thoroughly wash your hands, anus, and any toys you might introduce into your play. If you're into rimming, or there's the slightest chance of rimming, gently wash your anus, slightly inside and all over outside, with soap and water. Gargling with Listerine and showering with a mild soap postanal play has been shown to help rinse off and lower the risk of certain STIs.

## SHOULD I TELL?

A number of my patients ask me if they need to disclose their STI status to partners or hookups. If you have an active infection, yes. We are a community, and we need to be able to count on each other. It's not a fun call to make, but it's nothing to be ashamed of, either, and your partner(s) will likely be grateful that you cared enough to let them know so they can get evaluated and protect themselves.

Now, if you have herpes or HPV, but you've been treated and it's in remission, dormant, or inactive, and you're controlling the infection and taking your medicines, then whether or not you inform your Grindr hookup is an ethical decision I leave up to you. Obviously, if you have symptoms, like a cold sore, you shouldn't have ANY sexual or intimate contact with anyone until the symptom disappears. But unless they're symptomatic, most people wait until they find themselves in a relationship that seems to be getting more serious to disclose prior STIs.

However, should the status of your relationship(s) change, or you decide to no longer use protection, you need to be honest about your sexual history and vaccination status. Just lay all the truth on the table so that you can move the relationship forward and keep each other safe. And this is true no matter how you identify, what your sexuality is, or how you play.

————

So now you have a better idea why STIs are often referred to as "the gift that keeps on giving." I urge you to give yourself another gift—the gift of empowerment. Taking ownership of your ass and your health not only protects you, but also helps you protect your community. Be honest and commit to full disclosure to all your sexual partners. Society fails us time and time again by refusing to provide a thorough sexual education when we're young; let's not fail each other by keeping secrets and perpetuating stigma. Our community deserves proactive, thoughtful sex-care from our doctors, and from each other.

## CHAPTER 11

# Beauty Is in the Eye of the Buttholder

In 2023, we ran a nudity confidence survey. You know when most people said they felt confident about their naked bodies? During sex with the lights off. Yet think about the last time you had fantastic sex with a partner. Unless part of the fun was using blindfolds or otherwise not being able to see what you were doing, didn't you drink them in with your eyes *and* your mouth? Great sex is a feast for all five senses. Everyone deserves to be seen!

The majority of our survey respondents (82%) pointed to social media as the biggest source of pressure to conform to a certain aesthetic. It's a double-edged sword. On one hand, we're bombarded even more than previous generations by images of what we're told are standards of "perfection." By whom? Usually someone who wants to sell us something. On the other hand, social media can elevate and expose us to the widest variety of humans and their kaleidoscopic diversity of form, color, size, dress, hair, and yes, ass, the world has been able to see, ever. More of us need to expand our ideas of what we consider beautiful. Imagine the panoply of possibilities and experiences that could open up if we could shake off our preconceived ideas of what our ideal partners look like, and how freeing it would be for those of us who don't naturally fit into a culturally constructed mold. Imagine the mental energy (and money) we could devote elsewhere. It's certainly worth making the effort to expand our palates and repertoires.

But we are also sexual creatures, and the heart, not to mention all the other body parts, including the brain, wants what it wants. For people into anal, a fucked-up asshole, whether it really is one or they just believe it is, can be the equivalent of a fucked-up head. It can mess with your mind. It can impede your ability to connect, to de-stress, and to function. For many, expressing ourselves sexually is part and parcel of our mental and physical well-being. When we don't feel like we can do that freely and confidently, it takes a toll. This is why some of my patients are in despair by the time they get to me. They've gone to four or five anal surgeons asking to get an anal tag removed, or help with improving the look and feel of a scar following surgery, only to be told over and over their feelings aren't valid. To many doctors, if an imperfection doesn't hurt and isn't medically dangerous, it doesn't need attention. They'll even advise against touching it because "you'll only make it worse." That simply isn't true. So within reason, I'll do whatever it takes to help my patients achieve their ideal asshole (I don't perform Brazilian Butt Lifts (BBLs) or other procedures to enlarge or reshape buttocks, which are other popular aesthetic choices). People are already saddled with enough hangups that get in the way of them achieving their sexual and relationship potential; if I can ease even one, that's a win.

We can rail against the cultural conditioning that can lead people to believe they aren't perfect just the way they were born, but as one of my patients said, "There's nothing wrong with wanting to feel good about how your butt looks... When you get as much happiness and pleasure out of this part of the body as I do, [who's] to judge?"[1] The fact is, the perfect asshole is the one that makes you feel your sexy best. If it takes removing a skin tag to give you the confidence to feel like you could fuck on a brightly lit stage in front of ten thousand people at Madison Square Garden—or even just your partner in broad daylight—I'm all for it, and I'm glad I can help.

That said, I'm not interested in pushing some generic ideal. As a hole-centric doctor, I can vouch that everyone's asshole looks a little bit different, and all are beautiful. We've talked about how some imperfections and injuries can become sexual problems. When hemorrhoids, fissures, skin tags, or scars cause pain or restrictions, it's best to treat and fix them. But if they don't hurt or get in the way of your sex life, they may be just an aesthetic concern. And not everybody finds them off-putting. Some people thrill to the "rosebud" effect of rectal prolapse. Skin tags are totally subjective, too. I'll have a patient come in for a consult about another issue who'll tell me he has a huge skin tag that he wants me to leave alone, because even though he doesn't like it, his partner loves to bite and flick it. I'll have another patient come in specifically to talk to me about his tiny skin tag, adamant that I remove it as soon as possible because it makes him feel insecure when his partners ask about it. To each their own.

But for some, their unhappiness with or anxiety about their perceived aesthetic shortcomings has an effect on their psyche, and hence on their sex life. And some caboose connoisseurs have the same beauty standards for their fanny as they do for their face, and are willing to spend the same amount of time and effort on it. For them, we've got solutions.

There's a select number of perceived imperfections that tend to preoccupy people: hairy assholes, buttne, dark holes, scars, and divots. Let me reiterate that these are all purely cosmetic issues, and no one should ever feel like if they don't do something about them, they're less beautiful or desirable. There is absolutely nothing objectively unseemly or unattractive about a butt with hair, or a few scars, or some dimpled divots. It's all about what makes you feel beautiful and confident. If you want them gone, let me tell you how to get them gone. Some of these treatment options will be best handled by professionals in a spa or clinical setting, but wherever possible I've included instructions and advice for treatments you can do at your convenience in the privacy of your home.

## UNWANTED HAIR

It's totally normal to have asshole hair, and there are lots of people who absolutely love it, on themselves and on their partners. Many people don't mind having hair back there, but aspire to keep it neat and tidy. If that's you, here's a pro tip: use a clipper, and don't trim the hair too close. The closer you shave, the more stubble and friction you're going to experience. If you keep any amount of hair, make massaging it with a small amount of specially designed pubic-hair oil part of your daily hygiene routine. It keeps your skin smooth, prevents ingrown hair, and softens the follicles and hair, which will help decrease any friction. It also usually smells really nice.

A large number of people who love anal, however, prefer the smooth, sleek look and feel of a hairless asshole. Aesthetic preferences aside, a bald bunghole actually has some advantages. First, though one theory for the existence of butt hair is that it prevents chafing, if you have a lot it can cause friction during intercourse, which spoils all the fun, as well as in your daily life when shitting, exercising, or just moving around. Second, our hair traps oil, sweat, and bacteria, which helps keep the area clean, but can also lead to a more pungent posterior.

You've got a few options for removing unwanted hair if that's your preference. Waxing, sugaring, and even hair removal creams like Nair can give you a nice, smooth initial result, but there's a risk of stubble, acne, or ingrown hairs, where instead of growing straight out of the follicle, the new hair bends in on itself, often causing a painful red bump or pus-filled pimple. All of these side effects are unsightly, but worse, they introduce friction and irritation to anal play. If you use these hair-removal products, make sure to go somewhere that specializes in these services. If you insist on doing these treatments at home, please don't make the mistake of using hair removal cream in your butt crack unless you get off on feeling like you were recently skinned alive. You know what? Even then, don't do it. You'll be sorry.

Likely because it's the cheapest option, many people who decide to start grooming their butts begin by shaving with a razor. Unfortunately, it's not only complicated—you need to be a yoga master to twist yourself into a position that allows you to see clearly and reach all the angles of your ass without slicing yourself open—it puts you at risk of ingrown hairs,[2] razor bumps, skin tags, and, thanks to microtears, herpes outbreaks and anal warts.[3] Those microtears can make your skin itch as they heal, and the hair that grows back after a razor shave can feel like pine needles. No bueno.

Laser hair removal by a trained aesthetician is more expensive than any of these options, but it also limits the possibility for complications. Despite some marketing promises, it's generally not permanent unless you've been doing it for a very long time, but it does lower the number of times per year when you have to think about grooming this particular part of you, and the hair that does grow back is finer and softer. It's especially effective if you start early in your butt-grooming life before years of shaving and the subsequent acne and scarring that usually follow take their toll. Laser hair removal is a service that can also dramatically reduce the inconvenience and panic that ensues when the person you've been fantasizing about for months is suddenly on their way to your place for some unexpected playtime, and you've got the Amazon jungle growing back there and no time to prepare (deforestation is bad unless it's between your butt cheeks).

The treatment works by generating a light that gets absorbed by the hair's pigment, which converts it to heat that burns away the existing hair and damages the hair follicle, preventing the hair from regrowing quickly. It doesn't hurt so much as feel like a rubber band snapping repeatedly on the skin, though your aesthetician should adjust the settings as they target different areas. For example, the area around your hole will be more sensitive than the thicker flesh of the butt cheek.

Because the technology targets pigment, laser hair removal

was traditionally most effective for people with hair tones ranging from light brown to black, but recent improvements in technology now allow it to better accommodate a wider range of white, gray, light blond, and light red hair types. When hair color and skin tone are more similar, it might take longer to see results because the aesthetician has to work with a lower setting to avoid burning their patient. It's critical that you choose your laser hair removal clinic or medspa carefully. Only go somewhere that uses the most advanced laser technology that is safe for all skin types, that is staffed by properly trained laser technicians, and isn't squeamish about doing the procedure between the cheeks and close to the hole.

Taking the following steps and precautions before your visit will ensure your sessions go smoothly and prime you for optimal results:

1. Shave the area the 24–48 hours before your session. Wait a minute; didn't I just advise against shaving your butt? I did, but that's because hair grows back quickly after a regular shave. There are risks inherent in shaving with a razor, but they're not as likely when you're only doing it a few times per year, which is all that will be required once you start laser treatments, since you can go many weeks without needing to do it again. You have to get rid of the overgrowth of hair on the skin because the laser will be attracted to the hair's pigment, and if it burns the hair, it could also burn the skin.

2. Avoid exposing the area to the sun or tanning bed (no perineum sunning!).

3. Don't wax or pluck the area for one month prior to treatment.

4. Avoid taking antibiotics, or any medication that increases photosensitivity.

5. Don't use any products that may increase your skin sensitivity for one week prior to treatment, such as retinols, salicylic acid, benzoyl peroxide, or glycolic acid.

6. Don't use self-tanning lotion in the area being treated.

All of your hair doesn't grow at the same time—many follicles will be in a resting state when you get treatments—so in general, it takes about six sessions about one to two months apart to see a significant reduction in hair growth. Older people will see results in less time than younger patients still raging with hormones, but ultimately the speed at which the treatments work will be determined by the amount of hair you start with, your hair color, skin tone, pain tolerance, and schedule. Regardless of your coloring and hair type, an experienced aesthetician should be able to suggest appropriate guidelines and treatment during your initial consultation.

Some people who don't want to remove all their body hair, but do want to minimize friction between their cheeks, fear it'll look weird for their ass and only their ass to be smooth as a cue ball. Not a problem. Laser treatment can also be used to simply thin the hair for a natural look. This is an especially good idea for people with chronic irritation and those who shave or trim a lot, which causes microtears and stubble.

The following aftercare instructions should help keep you comfortable after your session.

1. You may see pink or reddish bumps for a day or so. This will fade, and your skin should regain its natural color and texture shortly following your hair removal session.
2. Avoid sun exposure for two weeks (once again, no perineum sunning).
3. Avoid friction and excessive heat to the treated area for at least eight hours.
4. Don't exfoliate your skin or use products that may cause irritation for several days after.
5. Resume moisturizing the area to keep hydration levels optimal twenty-four hours posttreatment.

## BUTTNE

We'd all like to think that, right along with curfews and mean girls, we'll leave acne behind once we age out of our teen years, but no. Year after year, zits linger like an unwelcome ex. And not only on our face! Tight clothes, exercise and sweat, excessive wiping, and even the wrong bodycare products can trap bacteria onto the skin of our ass. If the buildup starts clogging pores and hair follicles, they can get infected, causing what we doctors call folliculitis, and what everyone else calls buttne.

You can go a long way toward preventing buttne by showering, thoroughly drying your skin, and changing into a clean pair of underwear immediately after you work out or have sex. Incidentally, this also helps prevent swamp ass, that soupy, smelly funk caused by excessive moisture getting trapped between your butt cheeks. If you like to remove all the hair down there, including the butt cheeks, and laser treatments aren't an option or you prefer to wax, sugar, or shave, a butt facial, performed at the spa, can help prevent ingrown hairs. If you're susceptible to breakouts, a spa butt facial can help with that, too. And for everyone else who likes their hirsute state and just wants to keep their heinie as fresh as their face, a butt facial just feels nice. It should include extractions where necessary, as well as a deep cleanse, exfoliation, and hydration with moisturizers and serums. Some will even include a massage and a mask!

You can keep buttne away with at-home treatments as well. Use a bidet to keep from having to wipe too frequently, which darkens skin and can cause microabrasions. Scrubbing your ass a few times per week with an exfoliant specially made for the delicate anal area that both scrubs (exfoliating beads should be small and not too abrasive) and moisturizes will help keep cells rejuvenating and prevent clogged pores and follicles. And don't use a washcloth or mesh sponge—massaging the product into your skin with your hands will do just fine.

If you use silicone lube, exfoliate post-play to make sure you get it all off. Use products with gentle ingredients. You can add a soothing moisturizer after your shower to keep your skin smooth and supple. Choose something with anti-inflammatory and anti-itch ingredients (the one we make at Future Method has mango seed butter, jojoba, avocado oil, arnica flower, and echinacea). Above all, make sure whatever you use is very quick-drying. You don't want any moisture lingering between your cheeks that could promote the growth of bacteria or fungus. Make sure your skin is perfectly dry before getting dressed. Don't scrub with your towel! Pat yourself gently dry, and maybe build a little time into your morning to give your ass a few minutes al fresco. Enjoy being naked, especially in summertime. If you can spend the day at home, go commando under loose-fitting clothes. While you're at it, take a moment to check your fabulous self out in the mirror and give yourself some love. You deserve it, you beautiful thing.

## DARK HOLES

While every part of the body can be an erogenous zone, there's no doubt the darker colored bits are frequently where the magic happens. Nipples, genitals, ass—they're all a few shades darker than the rest of you. And there is absolutely nothing unsightly about that. Yet once porn stars started bleaching their butts, the anal community and people who love thong bikinis started clamoring for the service, too. Today anal bleaching is so mainstream[4], people of every skin tone consider it just another part of their beauty regimen.

**TOP TIP:** Anal bleaching isn't just for bottoms, it's for everybody's bottom! Sex is a pretty revealing sport, so by all means, if it makes you feel more confident or sexy to try lightening your hole, or trying any of the treatments discussed in this chapter, go for it! Think of all the years of pooping and sweating and working out that have built up. Over time, discoloration and changes do happen. People shave and trigger a case of acne. Scars can make the surface irregular or discolored. It's not just people who love to take or give dick in ass who take advantage of these cosmetic procedures. Many people find it feels good to freshen things up down there.

I prefer to refer to anal bleaching as "anal pigment lightening," or "anal fading" because there's no bleach involved in the process at all. It's actually a chemical peel designed to lighten the skin tone of the anus so that it blends in with the surrounding flesh, revealing less of a transition between butt cheek and hole. In some cases, it can help soften the look of scars, too. And some people discover after removing their hair for the first time that the hole and skin underneath is blotchy or otherwise.

For people who aren't looking for drastic change, an at-home cream treatment may deliver the results they want, though for best results, the process should be managed by a professional. It's a multistep procedure that generally begins at home, with the patient applying a pretreatment of topical hydroquinone 4% cream over the area they want to lighten for two weeks before their in-office appointment. The cream primes the tissue so it responds well to a hydroquinone chemical peel. During the office appointment, which will take forty-five minutes to an hour, the aesthetician applies the chemical peel. At the end of the appointment, the patient leaves still wearing the chemical peel, with instructions to shower it off eight to ten hours later. Starting twenty-four to forty-eight hours after the peel is removed at home, they'll repeat the nightly pretreatment of topical hydroquinone 4% cream for another two weeks. During this time, patients might report dryness, itchiness, redness, tightness, or discoloration over the treated area of skin, but that can be easily soothed with protective ointments like Aquaphor or Vaseline. For best results, the patient will return for a second in-office peel at the end of the two-week period.

Some patients with drastic hyperpigmentation may see their skin lighten by four to five shades, while others with less pigment may only see it lighten by one to two shades. In the early days, formulas could be harsh and cause chemical burns, but we've come a long way since then, and now, aside from perhaps some mild dryness and itching for a few days post-peel, there's no discomfort or negative side effects to the procedure.

## SCARS AND DIVOTS

A number of my patients who opt for anal pigment lightening first come to me for help with getting rid of old scars, often resulting from poorly healed fissures and hemorrhoid surgeries. Sometimes the scars are fine; sometimes they can be thick, raised, and pink (hypertrophic). They can be made less noticeable with a nonsurgical technique called microneedling that takes advantage of and ramps up the body's natural wound-healing process. Microneedling is performed with a tool that looks something like a thick pen, except instead of different colors of ink, the medical-grade tip contains dozens of needles. The aesthetician will glide the needles across the existing scar while they rapidly puncture the tissue at controlled depths with an up-and-down motion a bit like the needle on a sewing machine, essentially causing new micro-injuries. This breaks down the scar tissue and also induces your body to produce more collagen, a protein that plumps up youthful skin, but also helps skin heal when it's been damaged. For best results, it's important for microneedling to be done as early as possible during the postsurgical healing phase.

Patients are numbed with a topical cream like lidocaine in

advance of the procedure for comfort. The pain level is often described as being similar to getting a tattoo. Expect some mild bleeding from the tiny punctures in the skin. Afterward, you may see some peeling at the treated site, which is normal. It generally takes multiple sessions spaced four to six weeks apart for optimal results.

Sometimes microneedling to soften the appearance of scars doesn't work as well on people with darker pigmented skin, so we'll turn to anal pigment lightening as well, sometimes even tattooing the region with a matching color.

I also see post-surgery patients who complain about the appearance of divots or other irregularities in their butts, caused when a scar contracts, causing the skin to sink because it doesn't have any support. Others develop scarring or muscle atrophy that forms a ridge or step; this ridge or step then creates a functional problem by actually catching toys or dick upon penetration, causing tearing and pain. I'm still in an experimental stage with this treatment, but I've found that adding a little filler (I prefer Juvéderm products) can plump up the area and add symmetry, helping smooth away any perceived imperfections, plump up the space, and even lay down a kind of lattice that your body reacts to by refilling the space with native tissue as the artificial filler dissipates.

## AUGMENTATION

I don't perform butt augmentation surgery, but the demand is high thanks to the popularity of certain social media influencers and performers with particularly curvy buttocks. Procedures like butt implants, in which a silicone implant is inserted into or under the gluteal muscle, and fat grafting (commonly called Brazilian Butt Lifts, or BBLs), in which liposuctioned fat taken from other parts of your body are injected into your buttocks, have become extremely popular techniques for creating a fuller, rounder look. Unfortunately, too many people are allowing unqualified practitioners to perform these procedures on them. I've heard of people with limited budgets going overseas where the cost is cheaper, or turning to friends for injectables. In one case, a Florida-based unlicensed "toxic tush doctor"[5] injected a mix of cement, mineral oil, and flat-tire sealant into the bodies of people looking for affordable alternatives to getting the procedure done by a licensed practitioner. One of the patients died.[6] No matter what procedures you decide to try, but especially if you set your sights on something as invasive as plastic surgery, make sure you seek out licensed practitioners and board-certified plastic surgeons with reputable practices and extensive experience. You deserve the best.

## YOU'RE BEAUTIFUL. PERIOD.

The better we feel about ourselves—inside and out—the better our lives become, both inside and outside the bedroom. For some, the formula for fuckability can be found in a cream, filler, or scrub. For others, it's the right pair of underwear. It's not shallow to care about or enhance the way you look to please a partner, so long as the main person you're pleasing is yourself. We all want pretty, lickable, playable, pleasurable, and enjoyable assholes. You want to look like a porn star? By God, you should get to look like a porn star. And if you don't want to bother, you shouldn't have to. Self-acceptance is always one of our most beautiful features. Do what you want, just do it safely and with joy. Life is too short to sacrifice any part of our sexuality, or to compromise our deepest desires.

———

The most important beauty tip I can share with you is this: Love yourself. Love being you. Love being gay or straight, cis or trans. Love being not sure, if that's where you are. Love your ass, and love that you love ass. And if there's something about your ass you think could use some cosmetic improvement, love knowing that the solutions are out there. I promise, the secret to sexiness, and even happiness, is loving yourself and relishing every step you get to take on this exciting journey.

# Conclusion

About two years ago, a new patient—gay, married, age 63—sat in my office and wept. He'd come to me wanting to learn how to fuck. In his words, he was "desperate to learn how," "humiliated" that he didn't know, and "scared" of his own body.

He hadn't had penetrative sex since 1987.

Not long ago, he sent me a note chronicling his progress. The man who'd believed that masturbation was a form of cheating on his spouse was now pleasing himself weekly—and telling his husband about it at the dinner table, which frequently led to a round of lovemaking. He'd invested in dilators to keep his hole well trained, and various toys to enhance his pleasure. He felt seen by his husband, and understood his newfound sexual awakening as a "beautiful, sensuous exercise in mindfulness, alertness, and presence." I can't tell you how many of my patients come in for a procedure or aesthetic treatment and walk out hollering, "I should have done this years ago!" It's never too late to make a new start.

The path my patient followed was his own, but the process that led to his success was the same one I had to create for myself, and that now I prescribe for you. It starts with freeing yourself from everybody else's rules and expectations about what and whom you should want, and accepting who you are fully and without reservations. It starts with reveling in the fact that your body is built for pleasure, and that there is nothing shameful or dirty about indulging in every incredible sensation it has to offer, and that you have to offer others. It starts with taking the time to get to know your body intimately so that you can teach partners and loved ones how to treat it right, and so you can troubleshoot if things don't feel good. Let me take this moment to remind you that it's always supposed to feel good!

It starts but definitely doesn't end with using what you've learned in this book to continue exploring your sexual horizons, no matter who you are, how old you are, or how you identify. Tune in to your body-mind connection, and treat your body gently and kindly through healthy food and robust nutrition. Eat right so you feel good and are better able to make your partners feel good. Educate yourself so you know how to soothe your body when it hurts, pamper it to make it feel sexy and beautiful, and seek professional help when necessary. And let's take care of each other. Insecurity and fear breed dangerous behavior and bad decisions; you can lead others to anal bliss from a place of confidence, strength, and knowledge.

Bottoms, keep your hole well trained and warmed up with regular dilation so you can enjoy spontaneous sex when the moment strikes, and all sex with ease. Tops, share your knowledge with your partner(s) so that everyone's anal experiences are memorable for all the right reasons (I'm sure someone known as a Bottom Whisperer will find themselves in high demand). Experiment with positions. Try new toys. Open yourself up to the possibility that you can't know for sure what you do and don't like until you try it, so try everything that piques your curiosity. Good anal doesn't always come naturally, but is rather, like all beautiful forms of expression, communication and sensuality, an art and a skill. Enjoy the practice sessions!

There are people who will object to this book's existence, who will say that it's dangerous. But the real danger is ignorance. We have fully grown adults walking around who don't know their bodies and don't know where to turn for information. It's no wonder so many people get hurt or sick, physically and emotionally, as they try to discover more about their sexual selves. But newcomers, latecomers, and all cummers to this tribe, you now have the knowledge, the tools, and the step-by-step instructions to take you wherever you want to go in your sexual evolution, safely and joyfully. It's a great time to be a sexual creature. To be human. To be alive.

I hope you'll carry the celebratory message of this book out into the world with you. Let's work together to normalize conversations about sex—all kinds of sex. Let's make it a priority to create an environment in which no one ever has to be nervous going to see a healthcare professional, worried that they'll be faced with blank stares or worse, judgment, if they try talking about their sex life. Everyone deserves to be seen and to be understood. *You* deserve to be seen and understood. You can bet your ass that learning what you need to know to express your sexuality and create a fulfilling sex life will ultimately lead to better experiences and fulfillment in the other aspects of your life as well. Living and loving freely and fully without stigma, shame, or pain is truly the best medicine for us as individuals, for our community, and for future generations.

# Acknowledgments

How do I even begin to acknowledge all the individuals, institutions, and situations that got me to this point in my life—publishing my first fucking book! Cum on. And better yet, a book about fucking! Can't I just stop after bluntly thanking everyone that has an asshole or was an asshole or is still an asshole? I always say, "You learn more from observing what not to do in life."

But *I* would be an asshole if I didn't take the time to thank several important people for what has been a truly unbelievable journey thus far. First and foremost, my parents, Mel and Renee. Their unwavering love continues to this day and their own work—as dedicated New York City public school teachers—has allowed me to be in the same company of such amazing educators. They have taught me valuable lessons in how to write narratives and share knowledge that improves the lives of not only my community, but all communities. Then there's my older brother, David, his wife, Kristen, and their beautiful daughters, Brooke and Sienna, for their support in every step of my life.

I wouldn't be where I am today, nor specifically understand the way in which family plays a part in my existence, if I hadn't met my life partner, Andrew. His unconditional, unwavering love and commitment not only brought me out into the world, but also allowed me to accept, love, and live the life I was destined to live. Phoenix and Sebastian, my two beautiful boys, who truly, day in and day out, amaze me, let me rewrite the history of my own childhood once again. I still cry when thinking about the awesome responsibility taken and magnanimous gift given by both our egg donor, wherever you may be, and our surrogate mother, Heather, thanks to the advent of science and its modern marvels. It restores and reminds me that there are still kind and beautiful people in this fucked-up world. Ana, who makes our family's life that much better every single day, the kids are indebted to you, as am I. Neither my growth as a father or a human, nor this book, would have happened without your support. And thank you for allowing us to bring Oreo, our rescue dog, into our family. I am now officially a dog person.

The birth of Bespoke Surgical and all it has grown to become could not have been possible without Natasha and John, and then of course, the addition of Maxwell, Steve, Austin, and Tom. So much goes into this practice, and not just stemming from my consultation and surgical approaches. We have learned and grown so much as a team, making every patient's complex journey as simple and successful as possible. Same goes for the surgery centers, New York Center for Ambulatory Surgery and Midtown Surgery Center, in which I perform these operations. The staff that so professionally tends to our community's needs, becoming model allies, doesn't go unnoticed.

The best decision I ever made was to hire my dear colleague and now friend, Greg Lam—my go-to for absolutely everything. I would like to take the time to truly thank him and all his continued efforts. I was blessed to have him in New York for some time, where he met his now husband, Ari. Whether true or not, I take full responsibility for their meeting and consummation. Greg and I are seeing our dreams become reality through all our ventures, and I look forward to what the future holds. It's because of his hard work and dedication that Future Method, our product company that marries science and education with sex, was developed. The addition of David, our CMO, has continued our goal of taking over the world—one ass at a time.

When we discovered that people, and more so, doctors, weren't talking about anal sex and weren't asking the right questions specifically about gay sex, I knew we needed to make social and societal changes. Merritt, from mml pr, you and your team have been a godsend. We set out to change the world, making it a top priority to bring not only me and the practice to the forefront of sexual education, but also to truly start to take on sexual stigmas, removing the taboos and biases related to gay and anal sex. This daunting responsibility also comes upon the journalists in mainstream media outlets, all of whom have given us a platform to discuss important issues surrounding the sex ed no one ever received. The rebirth of this sexual revolution wouldn't have been possible without the current state of social media, and all of the influencers and their amazing followers, as well. Please all take a fucking bow!

Last, Michael, who listened to my anal ideas and then connected me with Will, my literary agent, who then got me in touch with Stephanie, without whom this book would never have been possible, and then Hannah and GCP Balance. Then to Boyking, the incredibly talented artist who took on the crucial role of turning my words on the page into cheeky and informative illustrations. I thank you all for trusting me and my vision, and for executing an anal bible that I hope will not only last for generations, but will also provide its readers with endless opportunities to enjoy all things anal.

I always tell people that I don't care what you shove up your ass. You should be able to do whatever you want, whenever you want, with whomever you want (of course, with consent)! And you should feel great about it. Love your body and your experiences. And if things go wrong, know the treatment algorithms and how to seek appropriate and affirming health care. I do believe that through this book, we have achieved our goal. And I say *we* because it took this anal army, including so many that I didn't have the space to list, to get to this point. It is a culmination of so many efforts, and I couldn't be any prouder to present to you, BUTT SERIOUSLY!

# Appendix A

## Anal Dilation Protocol Cheat Sheet

1. Choose a relaxing place. My favorite is the shower or bath. Make sure you have on hand your dilator set, a bottle of silicone lube, and a lube shooter (this last one is optional, but preferred).
2. Get into position. The best position for ensuring you get a direct hit when you insert your dilator is to stand upright or lie on your side if standing is difficult for you.
3. Clean the smallest dilator in your kit with soap and warm water, dry it with a lint-free towel, and cover it in lube. Use your fingers (make sure your nails are short and don't have any jagged edges) to coat the external skin of your hole, and then gently insert your lube shooter to insert lube deeper into your rectum and coat the sides of the anal canal. Keep your bottle of lube nearby; you're going to need more.
4. Insert the dilator into your rectum in an extremely gentle, slow, and smooth motion. You won't get very far before you feel resistance. Once you do, stop. Hold the dilator in place for three seconds before slowly removing it.

5. Repeat step 4, but first reapply lubricant to the dilator and apply new lube to the external anal area.

6. You will probably need to repeat this insertion, removal, and reinsertion four to six times before you're able to insert the dilator past all three muscles and fully into your hole. Remember: if you've chosen to use a dilator with a neck, "full insertion" ends before the neck. Don't ever push the dilator in past that point.

7. Once you've inserted your dilator that far, DO NOT take it all the way out. You're now going to pull the dilator back just a few centimeters each time before reinserting it all the way in. At this point you should always feel all three of your anal muscles engaging around the dilator.

8. Repeat this movement—only pulling the dilator back a few centimeters at a time, and never all the way out—twelve to fifteen times.

9. After completing your entire twelve to fifteen rep set, remove the dilator completely from your rectum.

10. Repeat the process—lubricating the skin and inner rim of your hole; lube shooting deep into the canal; lubricating the dilator; gently inserting the dilator; counting three seconds, retracting the dilator, and reinserting it until you can sink it all the way in. Once all your anal muscles are engaged around the dilator, leave it inserted while working it back and forth about twelve to fifteen times.

11. Once you're done, clean your dilator. Rinse it with water or wipe it with a damp paper towel or washcloth to remove any surface debris. Apply mild liquid body soap (if you're in the shower, you can use your body wash) and wash well for about

three minutes before rinsing with warm water. Once completely clean, place on a clean towel and air-dry completely before storing in a soft, safe place. If you're using a glass dilator, you can place it in the dishwasher on the disinfectant setting, or hand wash and then boil it for about three minutes in a pot of water.

12. You'll want to do two to three sets of the entire exercise, from initial lubrication to the twelve to fifteen rounds of constant muscle engagement, two to three times per week. Continue this routine for two weeks before moving on to the next size of dilator. Each session should only last for about three to five minutes. Give yourself a few days to recover in between each session.

# Appendix B

## Dilation Schedule

Week 1: Smallest dilator, two to three sets/wk (full insertion, twelve to fifteen rounds for muscle engagement)

Week 2: Smallest dilator, two to three sets/wk (full insertion, twelve to fifteen rounds for muscle engagement)

Week 3: Smallest dilator, one set, Medium dilator, two to three sets/wk (full insertion, twelve to fifteen rounds for muscle engagement)

Week 4: Smallest dilator, one set, Medium dilator, two to three sets/wk (full insertion, twelve to fifteen rounds for muscle engagement)

Week 5: Smallest dilator, one set, Medium dilator, one set, Large dilator, two to three sets/wk (full insertion, twelve to fifteen rounds for muscle engagement)

Week 6: Smallest dilator, one set, Medium dilator, one set, Large dilator, two to three sets/wk (full insertion, twelve to fifteen rounds for muscle engagement)

# Appendix C

## Directories for LGBTQ+ Affirming Medical Professionals

- https://www.lgbtqhealthcaredirectory.org/
- https://www.outcarehealth.org/outlist/
- https://www.glma.org/find_a_provider.php
- https://www.folxhealth.com/primary-care
- https://www.onemedical.com/
- https://www.apicha.org/
- https://www.lalgbtcenter.org/
- https://www.gaycenter.org/
- https://www.callen-lorde.org/
- https://www.thetrevorproject.org/
- https://www.bespokesurgical.com/

## LGBTQ+ Organizations

- SIECUS
- GLSEN
- Trevor Project
- HRC
- GLAAD

- SAGE
- Marsha P. Johnson Institute
- The Okra Project
- PFLAG
- National Queer & Trans Therapists of Color Network
- Transgender Law Center
- Transgender Legal Defense & Education Fund
- Lambda Legal
- Rainbow Labs
- Project Contrast

## Influencers to Follow

- https://www.instagram.com/sexwithashley/
- https://www.instagram.com/bybobbybox/
- https://www.instagram.com/gabriellekassel/
- https://www.instagram.com/thewright_rachel/
- https://www.instagram.com/sexedwithdbpodcast/
- https://www.instagram.com/sexwithemily/
- https://www.instagram.com/sexwithdrjess/
- https://www.instagram.com/dansavage/
- https://www.instagram.com/luvbites.co/
- https://www.instagram.com/drjoekort/
- https://www.instagram.com/joshuagonzalezmd/
- https://www.instagram.com/yourdiagnonsense/
- https://www.instagram.com/zacharyzane_/
- https://www.instagram.com/doctorcarlton/
- https://www.instagram.com/evyan.whitney/
- https://www.instagram.com/talk.tabu/

- https://www.instagram.com/gigiengle/
- https://www.instagram.com/lunamatatas/
- https://www.instagram.com/justinjlehmiller/

## Recommended Sex Shops

- Tom of Finland Store
- Circus of Books
- Hustler Hollywood
- Pleasure Chest
- Lovers
- Love Honey
- Good Vibes
- Babeland
- SheVibe

# Appendix D

## Foods That Are Rich in Soluble Fiber

- Black beans
- Lima beans
- Kidney beans
- Lentils
- Oats
- Flax seeds
- Sunflower seeds
- Chia seeds
- Hazelnuts
- Barley
- Edamame
- Brussels sprouts
- Sweet potatoes
- Broccoli
- Turnips
- Avocados
- Fruits like citrus (mostly in the peels), nectarines, apricots, carrots, guavas, pears, apples, strawberries, and, of course, peaches

# Notes

### Chapter 1

1. When my team surveyed: Dr. Evan Goldstein, "How Often Americans Have Anal Sex." *Bespoke Surgical*, October 29, 2019, https://futuremethod.com/blogs/the-future-edition/statistics-on-american-anal-sex-habits.

2. Meanwhile, "anal" consistently lands: PornHub, "2021 Year in Review," PornHub Insights, December 21, 2021, https://www.pornhub.com/insights/yir-2021; https://www.pornhub.com/insights/2022-year-in-review.

3. Armond and Dillon's workplace rimming session: Philip Ellis, The White Lotus Fans Have Some Notes on Armond's Subpar Rimming Technique." *Men's Health*, August 3, 2021, https://www.menshealth.com/entertainment/a37208935/white-lotus-hbo-rimming-scene-technique/.

### Chapter 2

1. Between 2006–2008, nearly half of men: Anjani Chandra, Ph.D. et al., "Sexual Behavior, Sexual Attraction, and Sexual Identity in the United States: Data from the 2006–2008 National Survey of Family Growth." *National Health Stat Reports* 36 (2011):1–36, https://pubmed.ncbi.nlm.nih.gov/21560887/.

2. The results from a 2015 anonymous survey: Alisa Hrustic, "Here's How Many Women Are Actually Having Anal Sex." *Men's Health*, Jul 28, 2017, https://www.menshealth.com/sex-women/a19527855/how-many-women-are-having-anal-sex/; D. Herbenick, J. Bowling, T.-C. Fu, B. Dodge, L. Guerra-Reyes, S. Sanders, "Sexual Diversity In The United States: Results From A Nationally Representative Probability Sample Of Adult Women And Men." *PLoS ONE* 12, no. 7 (2017), https://doi.org/10.1371

/journal.pone.0181198; K.L. Hess, E. DiNenno, C. Sionean, W. Ivy, G. Paz-Bailey, NHBS Study Group, "Prevalence and Correlates of Heterosexual Anal Intercourse Among Men and Women, 20 U.S. Cities." *AIDS and Behavior* 20, no. 12 (2016): 2966–2975, doi: 10.1007/s10461-016-1295-z.

3. In 2017, sex toy company Healthy and Active: "Are Men Finally Realizing Benefits of Prostate Massage?" Healthy and Active, September 19, 2017, https://www.healthyandactive.com/blogs/active-and-informed/are-men-finally-realizing-benefits-of-prostate-massage.

4. Thirty-seven percent of women in the 2015 survey: Hrustic, "Here's How Many Women."

5. In another survey taken in late 2021: Sean Jameson, "63.3% of Women Like Anal Sex." *Bad Girls Bible*, Dec. 23, 2021, https://badgirlsbible.com/do-women-like-anal-sex.

6. In a recent Indiana University survey: D.J. Hensel, C.D. von Hippel, C.C. Lapage, R.H. Perkins, "Women's Techniques for Pleasure from Anal Touch: Results from a U.S. Probability Sample of Women Ages 18–93." *PLoS ONE* 17, no. 6 (2022): https://doi.org/10.1371/journal.pone.0268785.

7. In 2020, the UK-based online sex toy retailer: Serena Smith, "How Young Women Feel About Pegging Their Boyfriends." *Refinery29*, Last Updated July 3, 2021, https://www.refinery29.com/en-gb/2021/07/10542856/my-boyfriend-wants-me-to-peg-him.

8. Almost a quarter of whom identify as straight: Jack Harrison, "Wonky Wednesday: Trans People and Sexual Orientation." *National LBGTQ Task Force*, June 5, 2013, https://www.thetaskforce.org/news/wonky-wednesday-trans-people-and-sexual-orientation/.

9. sex preferences are as varied: Ana Valens, "Trans/Sex: Here's What You Need to Know Before Having Sex With a Trans Woman." *Daily Dot*, March 22, 2019, https://www.dailydot.com/irl/trans-sex-myths-sex/.

10. How deeply they've embraced traditionally heteronormative: James P. Ravenhill, Richard O. de Visser, "'It Takes a Man to Put Me On the Bottom': Gay Men's Experiences of Masculinity and Anal Intercourse." *Journal of Sex Research* 55, no. 8 (2018): 1033–1047, doi:10.1080/00224499.2017.1403547.

11. Who can typically take over a decade: Ravenhill, de Visser, "'It Takes a Man to Put Me on the Bottom."

*Chapter 3*

1. Anal shallowing: Samantha Cole, "The Science on Anal Pleasure Is In (But Not All the Way)." *Vice*, June 30, 2022, https://www.vice.com/en /article/qjkpn3/the-science-on-anal-pleasure-is-in-but-not-all-the-way.

2. In 2017, my team surveyed: Dr. Evan Goldstein, "Do Doctors Ask Patients the Right Sexual History Questions?" *Bespoke Surgical*, Dec. 17, 2017, https://bespokesurgical.com/2017/12/01/doctors-asking-patients-right -questions-sexual-history/.

3. Only half of all U.S. medical schools: Sarah Beebe et al., "The Lack of Sexual Health Education in Medical Training Leaves Students and Residents Feeling Unprepared." *The Journal of Sexual Medicine* 18, no. 12 (2021): 1998–2004, doi:10.1016/j.jsxm.2021.09.011.

4. So are STIs: Eric Harvey, J.D., "Sex Education Laws and Public Schools." *FindLaw*, Last reviewed July 26, 2023, https://www.findlaw.com/family /reproductive-rights/sex-education-in-schools.html#:~:text=There%20are %20many%20studies%20showing,rates%20of%20STDs%20or%20STIs.

5. Incidents of sexual violence: Jo Yurcaba, "Sex Ed That Excludes LGBTQ+ People Is Tied to Worse Health Outcomes." *Forbes*, October 14, 2020, https://www.forbes.com/sites/joyurcaba/2020/10/14/sex-ed-that-excludes -lgbtq-people-is-tied-to-worse-health-outcomes/?sh=591b040b13cb.

6. Drugs and alcohol use: Hannah Slater, "LGBT-Inclusive Sex Educa- tion Means Healthier Youth and Safer Schools." *Cap20*, June 21, 2013, https://www.americanprogress.org/article/lgbt-inclusive-sex-education -means-healthier-youth-and-safer-schools/.

7. Many young people: Maureen Rabbitte, "Sex Education in School, are Gender and Sexual Minority Youth Included?: A Decade in Review." *American Journal of Sexuality Education* 15, no. 4 (2020): 530–542, https:// www.ncbi.nlm.nih.gov/pmc/articles/PMC7986966/.

*Chapter 4*

1. In one study: Jamie Ducharme, "Scientists Say This Popular Bathroom Accessory Really Does Help You Poop Better." *Time*, January 10, 2019, https://time.com/5498225/squatty-potty-study/.

2. There have been only a limited number of studies: Rena Goldman, "Squatty Potty: Does It Really Work and Is It Right For You?" *Healthline*, Updated

on December 23, 2021, https://www.healthline.com/health/does-the-squatty
-potty-work#how-it-works.

*Chapter 5*

1. "Off-screen pre-trial": Mark Hay, "Anal Sex in Porn is Much More Complex Than You Realize." *Vice*, May 16, 2017, https://www.vice.com/en/article/8qwkmg/how-to-do-anal-like-a-porn-star.

2. Up to two-thirds: Aurélien Garros, MD et al., "Risk of Fecal Incontinence Following Receptive Anal Intercourse: Survey of 21,762 Men Who Have Sex With Men." *The Journal of Sexual Medicine* 18, no. 11 (2021): 1880–1890, doi:10.1016/j.jsxm.2021.07.014.

3. Studies show these changes don't negatively affect: Richard E. Haaland et al., "Repeated Rectal Application of a Hyperosmolar Lubricant is Associated With Microbiota Shifts But Does Not Affect PrEP Drug Concentrations: Results From A Randomized Trial In Men Who Have Sex With Men." *Journal of the International AIDS Society* 21, no. 10 (2018): e25199, doi:10.1002/jia2.25199.

4. Nut allergies: Julia Wolov, "The Best Oil-Based Lubes for Long-Lasting Indulgent Sex." *Women's Health Interactive*, Updated July 2023, https://www.womens-health.com/best-oil-based-lube.

5. On the disinfectant setting: Bianca Alba, "How to Clean Sex Toys." *The New York Times*, June 10, 2021, https://www.nytimes.com/wirecutter/guides/how-to-clean-sex-toys/.

*Chapter 6*

1. Five-year study: Linda Searing, "The Big Number: Only 7% of Adults Are Consuming the Right Amount of Fiber." *The Washington Post*, June 21, 2021, https://www.washingtonpost.com/health/fiber-weight-control-heart/2021/06/18/2ff37134-cf7f-11eb-8cd2-4e95230cfac2_story.html.

2. FDA Recommended Daily Value: "Daily Value on the Nutrition and Supplement Facts Labels." U.S. Food and Drug Administration, Content current as of September 27, 2023, https://www.fda.gov/food/new-nutrition-facts-label/daily-value-new-nutrition-and-supplement-facts-labels.

3. That bulk helps "scrub" the sides of the intestines: "Why Fiber Is So Good For You." UCSF Benioff Children's Hospitals, https://www

.ucsfbenioffchildrens.org/education/why-fiber-is-so-good-for-you#:~:text =When%20you%20eat%20whole%20grains,your%20risk%20for%20colon %20cancer; https://www.mdanderson.org/publications/focused-on-health /how-fiber-helps-lower-your-cancer-risk.h11-1590624.html.

4. Hemorrhoids: "Eating, Diet, and Nutrition for Hemorrhoids." National Institute of Diabetes and Digestive and Kidney Diseases, last reviewed October 2016, https://www.niddk.nih.gov/health-information/digestive -diseases/hemorrhoids/eating-diet-nutrition#:~:text=Your%20doctor %20may%20recommend%20that,in%20your%20diet%20work%20better.

5. Decrease the risk of diverticulitis flareups: Barbara Gordon, RDN, LD and Esther Ellis, MS, RDN, LDN, "Diverticulitis." EatRight.org, reviewed January 10, 2023, https://www.eatright.org/health/health-conditions/digestive -and-gastrointestinal/diverticulitis.

6. Canned and frozen fruits and vegetables: Joy C. Rickman, Christine M. Bruhn, and Diane M. Barrett, "Nutritional Comparison of Fresh, Frozen, and Canned Fruits and Vegetables II. Vitamin A and Carotenoids, Vita-min E, Minerals and Fiber." *Journal of the Science of Food and Agriculture*, 2007, https://ucanr.edu/sites/kingscounty/files/19188.pdf.

7. According to the website: "Daily Value on the Nutrition," U.S. Food & Drug Administration, https://www.fda.gov/food/new-nutrition-facts-label /daily-value-new-nutrition-and-supplement-facts-labels.

8. General recommendation for fluid intake: "Nutrition and Healthy Eat-ing." *Mayo Clinic*, October 12, 2022, https://www.mayoclinic.org/healthy -lifestyle/nutrition-and-healthy-eating/in-depth/water/art-20044256 #:~:text=The%20U.S.%20National%20Academies%20of,fluids%20a %20day%20for%20women.

9. A well-hydrated body: Matthew Solan, "You Don't Say? The Many Col-ors of Urine." *Harvard Health Publishing*, May 1, 2022, https://www .health.harvard.edu/staying-healthy/you-dont-say-the-many-colors-of -urine.

10. Water-rich fruits and vegetables: "15 Foods That Help You Stay Hydrated." UCLAHealth, June 17, 2022, https://www.uclahealth.org/news/15-foods -that-help-you-stay-hydrated.

11. Bulk up your poo: Johnson W. McRorie, Jr. et al., "Psyllium: The Gel-Forming Nonfermented Isolated Fiber That Delivers Multiple

Fiber-Related Health Benefits." *Nutrition Today* 56, no. 4, 169–182, (2021): 169–182 *DOI:* 10.1097/NT.0000000000000489.

12. Fiber supplements affect every body: "Fiber Supplements Aren't One-Size-Fits-All, Study Shows." Stanford Medicine, April 28, 2022, https://med.stanford.edu/news/all-news/2022/04/fiber-supplements.html.

13. The composition of your microbiome: Doris Vandeputte, Gwen Falony, Sara Vieira-Silva et al.; "Stool Consistency is Strongly Associated With Gut Microbiota Richness and Composition, Enterotypes and Bacterial Growth Rates." *Gut* 65 (2016): 57–62, https://gut.bmj.com/content/65/1/57.

14. Acacia and psyllium husk: Kavita R. Pandey et al., "Probiotics, Prebiotics and Synbiotics—A Review." *Journal of Food Science and Technology* 52, no. 12 (2015): 7577–87, doi:10.1007/s13197-015-1921-1.

15. Researchers still aren't sure: "What Are Prebiotics and What Do They Do?" Cleveland Clinic, March 14, 2022, https://health.clevelandclinic.org/what-are-prebiotics/.

16. Research does indicate that they ease constipation and bloating: Maliha Naseer et al., "Therapeutic Effects of Prebiotics on Constipation: A Schematic Review." *Current Clinical Pharmacology* 15, no. 3 (2020): 207–215, doi:10.2174/1574884715666200212125035.

17. Synbiotics: Pandey, "Probiotics, Prebiotics."

18. Anal sex can promote a buildup: Adam Burgener et al., "HIV and Mucosal Barrier Interactions: Consequences for Transmission and Pathogenesis." *Current Opinion in Immunology* 36 (2015): 22–30, doi:10.1016/j.coi.2015.06.004.

19. When that booty biome is altered: David M. Phillips et al., "Lubricants Containing N-9 May Enhance Rectal Transmission of HIV and Other STIs." *Contraception* 70, no. 2 (2004): 107–10, doi:10.1016/j.contraception.2004.04.008; Pamina M. Gorbach et al., "The Slippery Slope: Lubricant Use and Rectal Sexually Transmitted Infections: A Newly Identified Risk." *Sexually Transmitted Diseases* 39, no. 1 (2012): 59–64, doi:10.1097/OLQ.0b013e318235502b; H. Rhodes Hambrick et al., "Rectal Douching Among Men Who Have Sex with Men in Paris: Implications for HIV/STI Risk Behaviors and Rectal Microbicide Development." *AIDS and Behavior* 22, no. 2 (2018): 379–387, doi:10.1007/s10461-017-1873-8.

20. Homosexual men are twice as likely: E. Mansoor, S.A. Martin, A. Perez,

et al.; "Epidemiology of Inflammatory Bowel Disease in Men With High-risk Homosexual Activity." *Gut* 72 (2023):1624–1625; "Gay Men Are Two Times More Likely to Have Inflammatory Bowel Disease, According to New Research." *The Daily*, September 15, 2022, https://thedaily.case.edu/gay-men-are-two-times-more-likely-to-have-inflammatory-bowel-disease-according-to-new-research/.

21. It can take anywhere from twenty-four hours: Elizabeth Rajan, M.D., "Digestion: How Long Does It Take?" *Mayo Clinic*, December 31, 2019, https://www.mayoclinic.org/digestive-system/expert-answers/faq-20058340#:~:text=All%20in%20all%2C%20the%20whole,days%2C%20depending%20on%20the%20individual.

22. As the intestines get irritated: Bárbara Frias and Adalberto Merighi, "Capsaicin, Nociception and Pain." *Molecules (Basel, Switzerland)* 21, no. 6 (2016): 797, doi:10.3390/molecules21060797; Kenneth Brown, M.D., "Why Eating Spicy Food Can Give You Diarrhea." *VeryWellHealth*, Updated on October 12, 2023, https://www.verywellhealth.com/why-does-spicy-food-cause-diarrhea-1088717#:~:text=Recap,This%20leads%20to%20diarrhea.

23. Even heavy coffee drinkers: Philip Ritchie, "Decaf Kills Coffee Withdrawal Symptoms." The University of Sydney, February 14, 2023, https://www.sydney.edu.au/news-opinion/news/2023/02/14/decaf-kills-coffee-withdrawal-symptoms.html#:~:text=Research%20conducted%20by%20the%20University,they%20knew%20it%20was%20decaf.

24. Sugar alcohols aren't rapidly absorbed: University of Maryland Medical System, "Top Reasons Sugar Alcohols May Not Be a Good Sugar Substitute." *Health. Wellness. Prevention.*, https://health.umms.org/2022/02/24/sugar-alcohols/#:~:text=The%20packaging%20of%20foods%20containing,can%20have%20a%20laxative%20effect.

*Chapter 7*

1. One of my patients: Client Tale, "Tales From the Tail—Guy Just Shat My Face!!!" *Bespoke Surgical, Medium*, December 17, 2019, https://medium.com/bespoke-surgical/tales-from-the-tail-guy-just-shat-my-face-3868696a569e.

2. "Poo water": Brian Moylan, "Gay Guys: You're Douching Wrong." *Vice*,

June 16, 2017, https://www.vice.com/en/article/59zq3x/gay-guys-youre -douching-wrong.

3. Suspect that douching can lead to higher incidences of HIV: Christian Grov et al., "Getting Clear About Rectal Douching Among Men Who Have Sex With Men." *Archives of Sexual Behavior* 50, no. 7 (2021): 2911–2920, doi:10.1007/s10508-021-01933-w.

4. STIs: Marjan Javanbakht et al., "Prevalence and Types of Rectal Douches Used for Anal Intercourse: Results From an International Survey." *BMC Infectious Diseases* 14, no. 95 (2014): doi:10.1186/1471-2334-14-95; M.T. Schreeder et al., "Hepatitis B in Homosexual Men: Prevalence of Infection and Factors Related to Transmission." *The Journal of Infectious Diseases* 146, no. 1 (1982): 7–15, doi:10.1093/infdis/146.1.7; Jerome T. Galea et al., "Rectal Douching Prevalence and Practices Among Peruvian Men Who have Sex with Men and Transwomen: Implications for Rectal Microbicides." *AIDS and Behavior* 20, no. 11 (2016): 2555–2564, doi:10.1007/s10461-015-1221-9; Henry J. C. de Vries et al., "Lymphogranuloma Venereum Proctitis in Men Who Have Sex With Men is Associated With Anal Enema Use and High-risk Behavior." *Sexually Transmitted Diseases* 35, no. 2 (2008): 203–8, doi:10.1097/OLQ.0b013e31815abb08; Heather Boerner, "Rectal Douching Injury in Men Who Have Sex With Men." *Medscape*, November 21, 2019, https://www.medscape.com /viewarticle/921697#vp_3.

5. Injuries: Grov, "Getting Clear About Rectal Douching."

6. Bowling pins and peanut butter jars: Kimberly Leonard, "They Got What Stuck Where?" *U.S. News*, June 10, 2016, https://www.usnews.com/news /articles/2016-06-10/they-got-what-stuck-where.

7. Condom use is dramatically lower than it used to be: Fenit Nirappil, "Men Are Using Condoms Less, Even as Syphilis and Other STDs Surge." *The Washington Post*, November 23, 2022, https://www.washingtonpost.com /health/2022/11/23/stds-rise-chlamydia-syphilis-condom-use/.

8. Only around one-third of MSM: Winston E. Abara et al., "Prevalence and Correlates of Condom Use Among Sexually Active Men Who Have Sex With Men in the United States: Findings From the National Survey of Family Growth, 2002, 2006–10 and 2011–13." *Sexual Health* 14, no. 4 (2017): 363–371, doi:10.1071/SH16034.

9. 78 percent of the gay and bisexual men: A. J. Hunt et al., "Changes in Condom Use By Gay Men." *AIDS Care* 5, no. 4 (1993): 439–48, doi:10.1080 /09540129308258013 https://pubmed.ncbi.nlm.nih.gov/8110858/.

10. Multiple studies of men: Alex Carballo-Diéguez et al., "Rectal Douching Associated with Receptive Anal Intercourse: A Literature Review." *AIDS and Behavior* 22, no. 4 (2018): 1288–1294, doi:10.1007/s10461-017-1959-3.

11. The rectal microbiome of men who receive condomless anal sex: Colleen F. Kelley et al., "Condomless Receptive Anal Intercourse Is Associated with Markers of Mucosal Inflammation in a Cohort of Men Who Have Sex With Men In Atlanta, Georgia." *Journal of the International AIDS Society* 24, no. 12 (2021): e25859 https://doi.org/10.1002/jia2.25859; Camilla Ceccarani et al., "Rectal Microbiota Associated With *Chlamydia trachomatis* and *Neisseria gonorrhoeae* Infections in Men Having Sex With Other Men." *Frontiers In Cellular and Infection Microbiology* 9 (2019): https://doi .org/10.3389/fcimb.2019.00358.

12. In a 2018 study of MSM: Alex Carballo-Diéguez et al., "Rectal Douching Associated with Receptive Anal Intercourse: A Literature Review," *AIDS and Behavior* 22, no. 4 (2018): 1288–1294, doi:10.1007/s10461-017-1959-3.

*Chapter 9*

1. Regularly resorts to using amyl nitrite (poppers): Austin Le et al., "Use of 'Poppers' Among Adults in the United States, 2015–2017." *Journal of Psychoactive Drugs* 52, no. 5 (2020): 433–439, doi:10.1080/02791072.2020 .1791373.

*Chapter 10*

1. The 2021 CDC analysis: Centers for Disease Control and Prevention: "Incidence, Prevalence, and Cost of Sexually Transmitted Infections in the United States." NCHHSTP Newsroom, last reviewed March 16, 2022, https://www.cdc.gov/nchhstp/newsroom/fact-sheets/std/STI-Incidence -Prevalence-Cost-Factsheet.html#:~:text=CDC's%20latest%20estimates %20indicate%20that,in%20direct%20medical%20costs%20alone.

2. According to the CDC: Centers for Disease Control and Prevention, "Incidence, Prevalence, and Cost."

3. PrEP doesn't prevent against other: Centers for Disease Control and

Prevention, "Continuing PrEP." HIV, Page last reviewed June 6, 2022, https://www.cdc.gov/hiv/basics/prep/continuing-prep.html#:~:text=PrEP %20provides%20protection%20from%20HIV,such%20as%20gonorrhea %20and%20chlamydia.

4. Almost half of the 26 million new cases: Centers for Disease Control and Prevention: "Incidence, Prevalence, and Cost of Sexually Transmitted Infections in the United States." CDC Fact Sheet, https://www.cdc .gov/nchhstp/newsroom/docs/factsheets/2018-STI-incidence-prevalence -factsheet.pdf.

5. Neurological and cardiovascular: World Health Organization, "Sexually Transmitted Infections, (STIs)." https://www.who.int/health-topics /sexually-transmitted-infections#tab=tab_1.

6. increased rates of various cancers: American Society for Microbiology, "The Dangers of Undiagnosed Sexually Transmitted Infections." December 8, 2022, https://asm.org/Articles/2022/December/The-Dangers-of-Undiagnosed -Sexually-Transmitted-In#:~:text=The%20Hidden%20Dangers%20of%20 Undetected,of%20cancer%20and%20HIV%20infection.

7. The number of new STI cases: Centers for Disease Control and Prevention: "Incidence, Prevalence, and Cost."

8. In some populations: Anne F. Luetkemeyer, M.D. et al., "Postexposure Doxycycline to Prevent Bacterial Sexually Transmitted Infections." *New England Journal of Medicine* 388 (April 2023):1296–1306 DOI: 10.1056/ NEJMoa2211934.

9. A preliminary study found that gargling with Listerine: E.P. Chow, B.P. Howden, S. Walker, et al., "Antiseptic Mouthwash Against Pharyngeal Neisseria Gonorrhoeae: A Randomised Controlled Trial and an In Vitro Study." *BMJ Journals* 93, no. 2 (February 2017): 88–93, https://sti.bmj .com/content/93/2/88.

10. It's estimated that between fifty to eighty percent of U.S. adults have it: Johns Hopkins Medicine, "Herpes: HSV-1 and HSV-2." https://www .hopkinsmedicine.org/health/conditions-and-diseases/herpes-hsv1-and -hsv2#:~:text=Herpes%20infections%20are%20very%20common,U.S. %20age%2014%20to%2049; Katharine J. Looker et al., "Global and Regional Estimates of Prevalent and Incident Herpes Simplex Virus Type 1 Infec-

tions in 2012." *PloS one* 10, no. 10, e0140765 (2015): doi:10.1371/journal.pone.0140765.

11. Even when successfully treated and healed: National Institutes of Health, "Why Genital Herpes Boosts the Risk of HIV Infection." August 17, 2009, https://www.nih.gov/news-events/nih-research-matters/why-genital-herpes-boosts-risk-hiv-infection.

12. Taking a daily preventative dose of valacyclovir: B.J. Anderson et al., "Prophylactic Valacyclovir to Prevent Outbreaks of Primary Herpes Gladiatorum at a 28-Day Wrestling Camp: A 10-Year Review." *Clinical Journal of Sport Medicine : Official Journal of the Canadian Academy of Sport Medicine* 26, no. 4 (2016): 272–278, doi:10.1097/JSM.0000000000000255.

13. 13 million new cases: Centers for Disease Control and Prevention: "Incidence, Prevalence, and Cost"; Kristen M. Kreisel et al., "Sexually Transmitted Infections Among US Women and Men: Prevalence and Incidence Estimates, 2018." *Sexually Transmitted Diseases*, 48, no. 4 (2021): 208–214, doi:10.1097/OLQ.0000000000001355; Harrell W. Chesson et al., "The Estimated Direct Lifetime Medical Costs of Sexually Transmitted Infections Acquired in the United States in 2018." *Sexually Transmitted Diseases*, 48, no. 4 (2021): 215–221, doi:10.1097/OLQ.0000000000001380.

14. Among MSM: Stephen Goldstone et al., "Prevalence Of And Risk Factors For Human Papillomavirus (HPV) Infection Among HIV-Seronegative Men Who Have Sex With Men." *The Journal of Infectious Diseases* 203, no. 1 (2011): 66–74, doi:10.1093/infdis/jiq016.

15. According to the CDC, at least four out of every five: Centers for Disease Control and Prevention, "Basic Information About HPV and Cancer." Last reviewed September 12, 2023, https://www.cdc.gov/cancer/hpv/basic_info/index.htm#:~:text=Usually%2C%20the%20body's%20immune%20system,and%20often%20has%20no%20symptoms; Mona Saraiya et al., "US assessment of HPV types in cancers: implications for current and 9-valent HPV vaccines." *Journal of the National Cancer Institute* 107, no. 6 (2015), djv086, doi:10.1093/jnci/djv086; Anil K. Chaturvedi, "Human papillomavirus and rising oropharyngeal cancer incidence in the United States." *Journal of Clinical Oncology: Official Journal of the American Society of Clinical Oncology* 29, no. 32 (2011): 4294–301,

doi:10.1200/JCO.2011.36.4596; Maura L. Gillison, "HPV Prophylactic Vaccines and the Potential Prevention of Noncervical Cancers in Both Men and Women." *Cancer* 113, no. 10 Suppl (2008): 3036–46, doi:10.1002/cncr.23764.

16. It's estimated that 90 percent of anal cancer: Aida Petca et al., "Non-sexual HPV Transmission and Role of Vaccination for a Better Future (Review)." *Experimental and Therapeutic Medicine* 20, no. 6 (2020): 186, doi:10.3892/etm.2020.9316.

17. Any number of things: Luigi Pisano et al., "Pap Smear in the Prevention of HPV-related Anal Cancer: Preliminary Results of the Study in a Male Population at Risk." *Giornale Italiano Di Dermatologia e Venereologia: Organo Ufficiale, Societa Italiana di Dermatologia e Sifilografia* 151, no. 6 (2016): 619–627, https://pubmed.ncbi.nlm.nih.gov/26199089/#:~+:text=Conclusions%3A%20Anal%20HPV%20testing%2C%20when,risk%20population%20targeted%20for%20screening.

18. Since its approval in 2006: Centers for Disease Control and Prevention, "Human Papillomavirus (HPV) Vaccination: What Everyone Should Know." Last reviewed November 16, 2021, https://www.cdc.gov/vaccines/vpd/hpv/public/index.html.

19. Incidence of anal warts in young AMAB: Donald G. McNeil, Jr., "HPV Vaccines Are Reducing Infections, Warts—and Probably Cancer." *The New York Times*, June 27, 2019, https://www.nytimes.com/2019/06/27/health/hpv-vaccine-warts-cancer.html.

20. At this time costs over $285.00 per shot: Gardasil.9 website, August 2023, https://www.gardasil9.com/adults/cost/.

21. One to two shots: World Health Organization, "One Dose Human Papillomavirus (HPV) Vaccine Offers Solid Protection Against Cervical Cancer." April 11, 2022, https://www.who.int/news/item/11-04-2022-one-dose-human-papillomavirus-(hpv)-vaccine-offers-solid-protection-against-cervical-cancer.

22. Forty percent of new cases: Centers for Disease Control and Prevention, "HIV Testing." Last reviewed June 9, 2022, https://www.cdc.gov/hiv/testing/index.html.

23. Decrease the risk of getting HIV: Centers for Disease Control and Prevention, "How Effective is PrEP?" Last reviewed June 6, 2022, https://

www.cdc.gov/hiv/basics/prep/prep-effectiveness.html; R.M. Grant, J.R. Lama, P.L. Anderson et al., "Preexposure Chemoprophylaxis for HIV Prevention in Men Who Have Sex With Men." *New England Journal of Medicine,* 363 (2010): 2587–99, doi: 10.1056/NEJMoa1011205; Kachit Choopanya et al., "Antiretroviral Prophylaxis for HIV Infection in Injecting Drug Users in Bangkok, Thailand (the Bangkok Tenofovir Study): a Randomised, Double-blind, Placebo-controlled Phase 3 Trial." *Lancet (London, England)* 381, no. 9883 (2013): 2083–90, doi:10.1016/S0140-6736(13) 61127-7.

24. Condoms alone reduce the risk of HIV to bottoms: Shaun Barcavage, NP, "How Well Do Condoms Protect Gay Men From HIV?" San Francisco Aids Foundation, October 17, 2016, https://www.sfaf.org/collections /beta/how-well-do-condoms-protect-gay-men-from-hiv/; Dawn K. Smith et al., "Condom Effectiveness for HIV Prevention by Consistency Of Use Among Men Who Have Sex With Men in the United States." *Journal of Acquired Immune Deficiency Syndromes* (1999) 68, no. 3 (2015): 337–44, doi:10.1097/QAI.0000000000000461.

25. Only a little over one-quarter of the U.S. population: Centers for Disease Control and Prevention, "PrEP for HIV Prevention in the U.S." Last reviewed September 29, 2023, https://www.cdc.gov/nchhstp/newsroom /fact-sheets/hiv/PrEP-for-hiv-prevention-in-the-US-factsheet.html.

26. In one controlled study: J. S. Keystone et al., "Intestinal Parasitic Infections in Homosexual Men: Prevalence, Symptoms and Factors in Transmission." *Canadian Medical Association Journal* 123, no. 6 (1980): 512–4, https:// www.ncbi.nlm.nih.gov/pmc/articles/PMC1704818/.

27. It's the most frequently: Walaa Elkholy et al., "Therapeutic and Prophylactic Effects of Punica Granatum Peel Extract Versus Metronidazole in Murine Giardiasis Intestinalis." *Journal of King Saud University-Science* 34, no. 8 (2022), https://doi.org/10.1016/j.jksus.2022.102321.

28. Entamoeba histolytica is another microscopic parasite: New York State Department of Health "Amebiasis (amebic dysentery)." Revised March 2023, https://www.health.ny.gov/diseases/communicable/amebiasis/fact_sheet .htm#:~:text=Amebiasis%20is%20an%20intestinal%20(bowel,stomach) %2C%20and%20weight%20loss.

29. Giardia frequently presents: T.B. Gardner and D.R. Hill, "Treatment

of Giardiasis." *Clinical Microbiology Reviews* 14, no. 1 (2001): 114–28, doi:10.1128/CMR.14.1.114-128.2001.

30. Entamoeba histolytica can cause amebiasis: Centers for Disease Control and Prevention, "Parasites-Amebiasis-Entamoeba histolytica infection." Last reviewed December 29, 2021, https://www.cdc.gov/parasites/amebiasis/general-info.html#:~:text=The%20symptoms%20are%20often%20quite,(poop)%2C%20and%20fever.

31. Both giardia and entamoeba histolytica: Gardner and Hill, "Treatment of Giardiasis."

32. Depending on the strain isolated: Centers for Disease Control and Prevention, "Parasites-Amebiasis-Entamoeba histolytica Infection."

33. Consistent use of condom: Christine M. Pierce Campbell et al., "Consistent Condom Use Reduces the Genital Human Papillomavirus Burden Among High-risk Men: The HPV Infection In Men Study." *The Journal of Infectious Diseases* 208, no. 3 (2013): 373–84, doi:10.1093/infdis/jit191.

*Chapter 11*

1. "There's nothing wrong with wanting": "Tales From The Tail: The New Approach to Anal Bleaching." *Bespoke Surgical*, April 1, 2020, https://bespokesurgical.com/2020/04/01/tales-from-the-tail-the-new-approach-to-anal-bleaching/.

2. Ingrown hairs: L. A. Brown, Jr., "Pathogenesis and Treatment of Pseudofolliculitis Barbae." *Cutis* 32, no. 4 (1983): 373–5, https://pubmed.ncbi.nlm.nih.gov/6354618/.

3. Herpes outbreaks and anal warts: Thomas W. Gaither, MD, MAS, et al., "Pubic Hair Grooming and Sexually Transmitted Infections: A Clinic-Based Cross-Sectional Survey." *Sexually Transmitted Diseases* 47, no. 6 (2020): https://escholarship.org/content/qt1k07p0tr/qt1k07p0tr_noSplash_fe4f90d51e851d471b5540edc00afc96.pdf?t=qeuxyu.

4. Anal bleaching is so mainstream: Ali Wentworth, "Anal Bleaching, G-Spot Enhancement, and the Lengths Some Women Will Go for the Ever-More-Perfect Body." *Marie Claire*, October 4, 2018, https://www.marieclaire.com/sex-love/advice/a712/anal-bleaching/.

5. A Florida-based, unlicensed "toxic tush doctor": DailyMail.com Reporter, "Transgender Woman Known as the 'Toxic tush doctor' For Injecting

Women's Buttocks With Silicone And Cement Is Sentenced To 10 Years Following The Death Of A Patient." *Daily Mail*, updated March 28, 2017, https://www.dailymail.co.uk/news/article-4355326/Transgender-woman -injected-cement-buttocks.html.

6. a mix of cement, mineral oil, and flat-tire sealant: Casey Glynn, "Report: More Women Claim Fake Fla. Doc Gave Them Cement Butt Injections." CBS News, November 22, 2011, https://www.cbsnews.com/news/report -more-women-claim-fake-fla-doc-gave-them-cement-butt-injections/.

# About the Author

**Dr. Evan Goldstein** is the leading anal health expert in the United States, founder of Future Method, and one of the few surgeons in the world whose practice, Bespoke Surgical, is dedicated to treating and restoring the human butt. He holds a perennial spot on the list of top doctors for the New York metro area, and *Crain's New York Business* listed him as one of their notable LGBTQ+ leaders and executives of 2020. He is frequently featured in national publications, is a popular podcast guest, and is in demand as a speaker for both medical and sex-positive industries. Well-known as a vocal advocate for the LGBTQ+ community, Dr. Goldstein is actively involved in a number of nonprofit organizations, including SIECUS: Sex Ed for Social Change, AIDS Community Research Initiative of America (ACRIA), and Human Rights Campaign (HRC). Dr. Goldstein lives in Katonah, New York, with his partner, Andrew, twin sons, and rescue dog, Oreo.